Your *Clinics* subscription just got better!

You can now access the FULL TEXT of this publication online at no additional cost! Activate your online subscription today and receive...

- Full text of all issues from 2002 to the present
- Photographs, tables, illustrations, and references
- Comprehensive search capabilities
- Links to MEDLINE and Elsevier journals

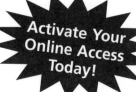

Activate Your Online Access Today!

Plus, you can also sign up for E-alerts of upcoming issues or articles that interest you, and take advantage of exclusive access to bonus features!

To activate your individual online subscription:

1. Visit our website at **www.TheClinics.com**.

2. Click on "Register" at the top of the page, and follow the instructions.

3. To activate your account, you will need your subscriber account number, which you can find on your mailing label (note: the number of digits in your subscriber account number varies from six to ten digits). See the sample below where the subscriber account number has been circled.

This is your subscriber account number

```
**************************************************3-DIGIT 001
FEB00   J0167   C7   (123456-89)   10/00   Q: 1

J.H. DOE, MD
531 MAIN ST
CENTER CITY, NY  10001-001
```

4. That's it! Your online access to the most trusted source for clinical reviews is now available.

theclinics.co

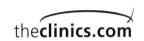

CLINICS IN
GERIATRIC MEDICINE

Elder Abuse and Neglect

GUEST EDITOR
Martin J. Gorbien, MD, FACP

May 2005 • Volume 21 • Number 2

SAUNDERS

An Imprint of Elsevier, Inc.
PHILADELPHIA   LONDON   TORONTO   MONTREAL   SYDNEY   TOKYO

W.B. SAUNDERS COMPANY
A Division of Elsevier Inc.

The Curtis Center • Independence Square West • Philadelphia, PA 19106-3399

http://www.theclinics.com

CLINICS IN GERIATRIC MEDICINE	**Volume 21, Number 2**
May 2005	**ISSN 0749-0690**
Editor: Maria Lorusso	**ISBN 1-4160-2647-9**

Reprints. For copies of 100 or more, of articles in this publication, please contact the Commercial Reprints Department, Elsevier Inc., 360 Park Avenue South, New York, New York 10010-1710. Tel. (212) 633-3813; Fax: (212) 462-1935; e-mail: reprints@elsevier.com.

The ideas and opinions expressed in the *Clinics in Geriatric Medicine* do not necessarily reflect those of the Publisher. The Publisher does not assume any responsibility for any injury and/or damage to persons or property arising out of or related to any use of the material contained in this periodical. The reader is advised to check the appropriate medical literature and the product information currently provided by the manufacturer of each drug to be administered to verify the dosage, the method and duration of administration, or contraindications. It is the responsibility of the treating physician or other health care professional, relying on independent experience and knowledge of the patient, to determine drug dosages and the best treatment for the patient. Mention of any product in this issue should not be construed as endorsement by the contributors, editors, or the Publisher of the product or manufacturers' claims.

Clinics in Geriatric Medicine (ISSN 0749-0690) is published quarterly by W.B. Saunders Company. Corporate and editorial offices: The Curtis Center, Independence Square West, Philadelphia, PA 19106-3399. Accounting and circulation offices: 6277 Sea Harbor Drive, Orlando, FL 32887-4800. Periodicals postage paid at Orlando, FL 32862, and additional mailing offices. Subscription price is $160.00 per year (US individuals), $260.00 per year (US institutions), $205.00 per year (Canadian individuals), $320.00 per year (Canadian institutions), $210.00 per year (foreign indi-viduals), and $320.00 per year (foreign institutions). Foreign air speed delivery is included in all *Clinics* subscription prices. All prices are subject to change without notice. POSTMASTER: Send address changes to *Clinics in Geriatric Medicine* W.B. Saunders Company, Periodicals Fulfillment, Orlando, FL 32887-4800. **Customer Service: 1-800-654-2452 (US). From outside of the US, call 1-407-345-4000. E-mail:hhspcs@harcourt.com.**

Clinics in Geriatric Medicine is covered in *Index Medicus*, *EMBASE/Excerpta Medica*, *Current Contents/Clinical Medicine (CC/CM)*, *and the Cumulative Index to Nursing & Allied Health Literature*.

Printed in the United States of America.

GUEST EDITOR

MARTIN J. GORBIEN, MD, FACP, Director, Section of Geriatric Medicine, Rush Department of Internal Medicine, Rush University Medical Center, Chicago, Illinois

CONTRIBUTORS

TIMOTHY BAKER, PhD, Data Integrity, Inc., West Newton, Massachusetts

ANN W. BURGESS, RN, DNSc, FAAN, Professor of Psychiatric Nursing, W.F. Connell School of Nursing, Boston College, Chestnut Hill, Massachusetts

ELAINE CHEN, BS, Rush Medical College, Chicago; and Senior Medical Student, Rush Medical College, Chicago, Illinois

CAMERON R. DEGUERRE, Law Clerk, Peck, Bloom, Austriaco & Mitchell, LLC., Chicago, Illinois; and May 2005 JD Candidate, DePaul University College of Law, Chicago, Illinois

XINQI DONG, MD, Instructor, Department of Medicine, Section of Geriatrics, University of Chicago, Chicago, Illinois

CARMEL B. DYER, MD, Associate Professor, Department of Medicine, Baylor College of Medicine, Houston; Director, Geriatrics Program, Baylor College of Medicine, Houston; and Co-Director, Texas Elder Abuse & Mistreatment (T.E.A.M.) Institute, Houston, Texas

AMY R. EISENSTEIN, MA, Education Coordinator, Section of Geriatric Medicine, Rush University Medical Center, Chicago, Illinois

JOSEPH H. FLAHERTY, MD, Associate Professor, Division of Geriatrics, Department of Internal Medicine, Saint Louis University School of Medicine, St. Louis; and Geriatric Research Education and Clinical Center, St. Louis VA Medical Center, St. Louis, Missouri

ANGELA M. GEROLAMO, RN, MSN, Pre-Doctoral Fellow, The Center for Health Outcomes and Policy Research, University of Pennsylvania School of Nursing, Philadelphia, Pennsylvania

MARTIN J. GORBIEN, MD, FACP, Director, Section of Geriatric Medicine, Rush Department of Internal Medicine, Rush University Medical Center, Chicago, Illinois

NANCY P. HANRAHAN, RN, PhD, Assistant Professor, Center for Health Outcomes and Policy Research, University of Pennsylvania School of Nursing, Philadelphia, Pennsylvania

MARIA R. HANSBERRY, MD, Department of Internal Medicine, Section of Geriatric Medicine, Rush University Medical Center, Chicago; and Assistant Professor, Department of Internal Medicine, Section of Geriatric Medicine, Rush University Medical Center, Chicago, Illinois

CANDACE J. HEISLER, JD, CJ Heisler & Associates, San Bruno, California

CARRIE A. HILL, BSW, Guardianship Specialist, Texas Department of Family and Protective Services; and Member, Texas Elder Abuse & Mistreatment (T.E.A.M.) Institute, Houston, Texas

SEEMA JOSHI, MD, Fellow, Division of Geriatrics, St. Louis University School of Medicine, St. Louis; and Geriatric Research Education and Clinical Center, St. Louis VA Medical Center, St. Louis, Missouri

LUCIA C. KIM, MD, MPH, Assistant Professor, Department of Medicine, Baylor College of Medicine; and Member, Texas Elder Abuse & Mistreatment (T.E.A.M.) Institute, Houston, Texas

RAY J. KOENIG III, JD, Senior Associate Attorney, Peck, Bloom, Austriaco & Mitchell, LLC., Chicago, Illinois

KATHLEEN QUINN, Past President, National Association of Adult Protective Services; and Former Director of the Illinois Elder abuse and Neglect Program, Springfield, Illinois

KIMBERLY REED, RN, JD, LLM, Attorney-at-Law, Registered Professional Nurse (BSN), Reed Law Associates, PC, Northbrook, Illinois

ANNE R. SIMPSON, MD, CMD, Associate Professor of Medicine, Division of Geriatrics, Department of Internal Medicine; Jack and Donna Rust Professor of Biomedical Ethics; and Director of the Institute for Ethics, The University of New Mexico Health Sciences Center, School of Medicine, Albuquerque, New Mexico

HOLLY ZIELKE, MA, Elder Abuse Program, Illinois Department on Aging, Chicago, Illinois

CONTENTS

Preface   xi
Martin J. Gorbien

Elder Abuse and Neglect: An Overview   279
Martin J. Gorbien and Amy R. Eisenstein

The dramatic growth of the American elderly population has great
implications for our health care system. The "demographic imperative" that has fueled the awareness of the needs of older adults
has a major impact on issues related to social welfare, justice, and
economics. There are 45 million people over the age of 60 and
3 million over the age of 85. Those over age 85 represent the fastest
growing segment of the elderly population. With this trend comes
a segment of the population that is at risk for abuse, neglect, or
self-neglect. We are challenged to be aware of the many faces of
elder mistreatment and to understand it in the broader context
of domestic violence. All health care professionals working with
older adults need to become familiar with the recognition, treatment, and prevention of elder abuse and neglect.

Medical Implications of Elder Abuse and Neglect   293
XinQi Dong

Health care professional's role in recognition of elder abuse and
neglect has been a relatively recent phenomenon. Millions of elderly
suffer as the result of abuse and neglect each year in the form of
worsened quality of life, higher health system utilization, and high
risk for mortality. Health care professionals are uniquely situated
in detecting, reporting, and managing suspected cases of elder abuse
and neglect, yet many barriers exist both on the individual level as
well as a broader need for system change. Through education, training and reinforcement, health care providers could be more involved
in providing effective management protocols and guidelines to advocate for our elders in the current epidemic of abuse and neglect.

Dementia and Elder Abuse 315
Maria R. Hansberry, Elaine Chen, and Martin J. Gorbien

Dementia and elder abuse are relatively common and under-
diagnosed geriatric syndromes. A unique relationship is observed
when the two entities coexist. Special issues can confound the care
of the dementia patient suspected of being abused. Impaired language or motor abilities to communicate abusive situations to a
third party, lack of decisional capacity to address the abusive situation, disinhibited behavior that contributes to a cycle of violence,
and coincident depression of the abused elder complicate the diagnosis and management of elder abuse. Education of the caregiver
and attention to caregiver stress, including depression, may prevent onset and perpetuation of abuse.

Elder Abuse and Neglect in Long-Term Care 333
Seema Joshi and Joseph H. Flaherty

Patient and caregiver education and other interventions targeted
toward risk factors or types of abuse or neglect play an invaluable
role in preventing elder abuse and mistreatment.

Cultural Issues and Elder Mistreatment 355
Anne R. Simpson

The article is a brief discussion of a few of the complex issues
that may represent a cultural component of elder mistreatment.
Reference is made to historical perspectives and subcultures. The
goals of the article are to broaden the discussion around the issues
of elder abuse in various population groups and to consider some
methods of intervention.

When Elders Lose their Cents: Financial Abuse of the Elderly 365
Kimberly Reed

Elder financial abuse is one of the most difficult types of elder
abuse to diagnose given its lack of overt physical symptomatology.
Unusual bank account activity, sudden changes of beneficiaries
or agents in estate planning or advance directive documents,
and worsening of medical conditions due to lack of follow-up or
unfilled prescriptions are indicators of potential financial abuse.
Federal laws are aimed at education and prevention (not treatment), whereas state laws are more comprehensive. Criminal and
civil legal remedies exist to bring the abuser to justice, but the emotional trauma of financial exploitation lasts a long time.

**The Legal and Governmental Response to Domestic
Elder Abuse**   383
Ray J. Koenig III and Cameron R. DeGuerre

> Older Americans constitute the fastest growing segment of the
> United States population and may account for 20% of the Unites
> States population by 2050. The federal government has taken mini-
> mal action to identify and solve their problems. Due to the federal
> government's inaction, states have become the primary engine for
> combating abuse. This is most often seen through adult protective
> services, which primarily consist of mandatory reporting laws, invol-
> untary interventions, and educational programs. Funding is the pri-
> mary roadblock to the successful execution of state laws targeting
> domestic elder abuse. The proposed federal Elder Justice Act of 2003,
> if passed, may fill in the gaps of current federal legislation by imple-
> menting a uniform method of response to domestic elder abuse and
> providing funding to the states to rectify instances of abuse.

Forensic Markers in Elder Female Sexual Abuse Cases   399
Ann W. Burgess, Nancy P. Hanrahan, and Timothy Baker

> Evidence exists that older adults are victims of sexual assault
> and rape. The scope of the problem, prevalence, and correlates of
> these sex crimes are relatively unknown. Such knowledge deficits
> are major barriers to detecting, prosecuting, and preventing sex
> crimes against older adults. Understanding how intentional sexual
> injuries are inflicted on older adults is a growing concern as the
> population over 65 increases. This study contributes critical infor-
> mation to guide the identification of physical and psychologic
> markers of elder sexual abuse to be integrated by clinicians and
> law enforcement as forensic medical evidence.

Core Data Elements Tracking Elder Sexual Abuse   413
Nancy P. Hanrahan, Ann W. Burgess, and Angela Gerolamo

> Sexual abuse in the older adult population is an understudied vec-
> tor of violent crimes with significant physical and psychological
> consequences for victims and families. Research requires a theoret-
> ical framework that delineates core elements using a standardized
> instrument. To develop a conceptual framework and identify core
> data elements specific to the older adult population, clinical, admin-
> istrative, and criminal experts were consulted using a nominal
> group method to revise an existing sexual assault instrument. The
> revised instrument could be used to establish a national database
> of elder sexual abuse. The database could become a standard
> reference to guide the detection, assessment, and prosecution of
> elder sexual abuse crimes as well as build a base from which pol-
> icy makers could plan and evaluate interventions that targeted
> risk factors.

Community Approaches to Elder Abuse   **429**
Carmel B. Dyer, Candace J. Heisler, Carrie A. Hill,
and Lucia C. Kim

> Collaboration of professionals from diverse disciplines is required
> to address the multiple, complex issues and needs of community-
> dwelling elders who are abused or neglected. Reporting suspected
> elder abuse or neglect cases to Adult Protective Service (APS)
> agencies provides access to services that address the social, med-
> ical, and legal needs of elderly persons. A geriatric interdiscipli-
> nary team can provide a comprehensive medical, functional, and
> social assessment. Based on the findings from the assessment and
> in collaboration with the APS team, the intervention plan can be
> formulated. Some cases of elder abuse or neglect may require
> intervention from the criminal justice or the civil justice system for
> serious legal issues such as sexual assault, financial exploitation, or
> guardianship. Other resources, such as Area Agencies on Aging,
> local women's shelters, and The National Center for Elder Abuse,
> are available to help manage elder abuse and neglect cases in
> the community.

Elder Abuse, Neglect, and Exploitation: Policy Issues   **449**
Kathleen Quinn and Holly Zielke

> Elder abuse remains a rapidly growing but largely invisible national
> policy issue. As the number of elderly persons increases, so will
> elder abuse, neglect, and financial exploitation. This has implica-
> tions not only for the victims and the programs struggling to pro-
> tect them but also for publicly funded programs such as Medicare
> and Medicaid. The urgent problem is to address elder abuse on a
> national level in a comprehensive and informed way to prevent the
> untold suffering of hundreds of thousands of older persons who
> deserve to live their final years with dignity and security.

Index   **459**

FORTHCOMING ISSUES

August 2005
Rheumatic Diseases in the Elderly
Arthur F. Kavanaugh, MD, *Guest Editor*

November 2005
Obesity
Suzanne Fields, MD, and
Lisa Strano-Paul, MD, *Guest Editors*

February 2006
Anticoagulation
Laurie Jacobs, MD, *Guest Editor*

PREVIOUS ISSUES

February 2005
Palliative Care II: Improving Care
Linda L. Emanuel, MD, PhD, *Guest Editor*

November 2004
Palliative Care I: Providing Care
Linda L. Emanuel, MD, PhD, *Guest Editor*

August 2004
Geriatric Incontinence
Margaret-Mary G. Wilson, MBBS, MRCP,
FNMCP, *Guest Editor*

CLINICS IN
GERIATRIC
MEDICINE

ELSEVIER
SAUNDERS

Clin Geriatr Med 21 (2005) xi–xiii

Preface

Elder Abuse and Neglect

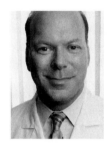

Martin J. Gorbien, MD, FACP
Guest Editor

The phrase *demographic imperative* is used frequently when discussing any topic relevant to the growing population of older adults. It is at the core of the burgeoning fields of geriatric medicine and gerontology. The number of people 85 and older will be seven times higher in 2050 than it was in 1980. In 2030, 20% of the population will be elderly. Experts in the field of aging urge governmental officials to allow the *demographic imperative* to appropriately effect public policy. This simple phrase takes on special meaning when we begin to discuss elder abuse and neglect. In the United States, the growing population of frail, vulnerable citizens throughout the community and in institutions has resulted in a daunting task of keeping this population safe and free from harm while respecting their autonomy. Many who have chosen careers working on behalf of this population were drawn to it because of the challenge of unmet needs of elders.

Age-related syndromes that result in frailty, functional decline, or psychiatric illness increase the risk of abuse, neglect, and self-neglect. We have been limited by a paucity of data and sound scientific research on this subject. A review of this field's brief history reveals progress in the study of elder abuse and response in legislation and programming. Legislation dealing with this form of domestic violence may vary significantly from state to state. More recently, there have been substantive changes at the national level to standardize our approach to the study of elder mistreatment. Ideally, an improved approach will lead to better programs devoted to the prevention and response to elder abuse and neglect.

Our best estimates indicate that between 1 and 2 million Americans over the age of 65 are mistreated each year [1]. Every report on the topic of abuse or neglect cautions us of the underrepresentation of its prevalence. The vexing discussion of self-neglect appropriately reminds us of how little we know about a subject even more difficult to define, identify, and remedy. The demographic imperative suggests that all of these problems will grow along with the population. The concept of unmet needs of this growing, at-risk older population remains at the center of the societal challenge.

The National Research Council's 2003 compendium provides a comprehensive summary of the history of the study of elder mistreatment, current data, and future research needs [2]. It is an important work and serves as an excellent resource for students and professionals interested in this subject. The extensive, interdisciplinary panel of experts reflects the importance of contributions from a vast array of fields.

"The test of a people is how it behaves towards the old." This famous quote by Abraham Joshua Heschel describes the importance of this critical, modern-day issue with clarity, elegance, and power. Elder abuse and neglect as well as self-neglect are public health issues. With the privilege of caring for any marginalized population comes the challenge of meeting their vast needs and protecting their interests.

This issue of the *Clinics in Geriatric Medicine* provides an update on a wide range of issues in the area of elder abuse and neglect intended to give clinicians and others a compendium of current information on this broad subject. The scope of elder mistreatment is great. The categories of mistreatment are diverse. Physical, sexual, financial, and emotional abuse can be very different entities despite their common root in domestic violence. The special relationship between dementia and elder mistreatment is fascinating and frightening given future projections for dementia cases in the United States. Team care will become even more essential. Physicians, nurses, and social workers will note that we need to call upon a diverse group of professionals to examine and respond to elder mistreatment in the comprehensive manner that it deserves. Health care professionals will succeed in their efforts on behalf of elder mistreatment by developing collaborative programs with representatives from law enforcement, financial, governmental, and legal entities. We are grateful to the authors for their scholarly treatment of topics that underscore the need for support for an interdisciplinary approach to vulnerable older adults.

It is with deep gratitude and great reverence that we acknowledge the pioneering and enduring work of the late Dr. Rosalie Wolf.

Martin J. Gorbien, MD, FACP
Section of Geriatric Medicine
Rush University Medical Center
710 S. Paulina Street
Chicago, IL 60612, USA
E-mail address: martin_gorbien@rush.edu

References

[1] Pillemer K, Finkelhor D. The prevalence of elder abuse: a random sample survey. The Gerontologist 1988;28(1):51–7.

[2] National Research Council. In: Bonnie RJ, Wallace RB, editors. Elder mistreatment: abuse, neglect and exploitation in an aging America. Panel to Review Risk and Prevalence of Elder Abuse and Neglect. Committee on National Statistics and Committee on Law and Justice, Division of Behavioral and Social Sciences and Education. Washington, DC: The National Acadamies Press; 2003.

ELSEVIER
SAUNDERS

CLINICS IN
GERIATRIC
MEDICINE

Clin Geriatr Med 21 (2005) 279–292

Elder Abuse and Neglect: An Overview

Martin J. Gorbien, MD, FACP*, Amy R. Eisenstein, MA

Section of Geriatric Medicine, Department of Internal Medicine, Rush University Medical Center, 710 S. Paulina Street, Chicago, IL 60612, USA

The dramatic growth of the American elderly population has great implications for our health care system. The "demographic imperative" that has fueled the awareness of the needs of older adults has a major impact on issues related to social welfare, justice, and economics. There are 45 million people over the age of 60 and 3 million over the age of 85. Those over age 85 represent the fastest growing segment of the elderly population. The number of people 85 and older will be seven times higher in 2050 than it was in 1980. In 2030, 20% of the population will be elderly [1]. With this trend comes a segment of the population that is at risk for abuse, neglect, or self-neglect [2]. We are challenged to be aware of the many faces of elder mistreatment and to understand it in the broader context of domestic violence. All health care professionals working with older adults need to become familiar with the recognition, treatment, and prevention of elder abuse and neglect.

Background

Elder abuse was recognized in ancient societies. In *Old Age*, de Beauvior analyzes Roman literature, which often describes its elders with derision and loathing [3]. King Lear's message to his daughter Cordelia, "I am mightily abused. I should even die with pity…." is Shakespeare's reflection of one regrettable father–daughter relationship [4]. In Jonathan Swift's *Gulliver's Travels*, the poverty and isolation of those over 80 is poignantly depicted and often quoted in gerontology classes [5].

---

* Corresponding author.
E-mail address: mgorbien@rush.edu (M.J. Gorbien).

0749-0690/05/$ – see front matter © 2005 Elsevier Inc. All rights reserved.
doi:10.1016/j.cger.2004.12.001

geriatric.theclinics.com

Modern reports of elder abuse were first noted in the medical literature in England in 1975 when the *British Medical Journal* published a report of "granny battering" [6]. In the United States in the 1950s, Congress developed financial incentives for states to develop protective service programs, although cost and efficacy were questioned. Reports of abuse and neglect in nursing homes in the 1970s made way for a more systematic study of elder mistreatment as a result of a United States Senate Special Committee on Aging [7]. The 1981 United States House of Representatives Select Committee on Aging allowed victims of elder abuse to share personal testimony. The committee reported that "elder abuse is far from an isolated and localized problem involving a few frail elderly and their pathological offspring. The problem is a full-scale national problem which exists with a frequency which few have dared to imagine. In fact, abuse of the elderly by their loved ones and caretakers exists with a frequency and rate only slightly less than child abuse on the basis of the data supplied by the States" [8]. However, a federal elder abuse act failed to pass in that same year. Throughout the early 1990s, there was much activity at the national level as a result of the United States Department of Health and Human Services' Elder Abuse Task Force and the creation of the National Institute on Elder Abuse. Despite the ongoing limitations of research in the area of elder mistreatment, the last decade represents a period of significant progress [9].

Defining elder abuse

Defining elder abuse and neglect has been influenced by governmental agencies and by researchers. The 1985 Elder Abuse Prevention, Identification and Treatment Act defined abuse as the "willful infliction of injury, unreasonable confinement, intimidation or cruel punishment with resulting physical harm or pain or mental anguish, or the willful deprivation by a caretaker of goods or services which are necessary to avoid physical harm, mental anguish or mental illness" [10]. Other definitions have been more needs oriented and tend to replace the terms "abuse" and "neglect" with the concept of the caregiver's inability to meet the needs of the older adult or mistreatment of the older adult. Thus, acts of omission and commission are acknowledged. These definitions are less criminally oriented and therefore are less likely to create stigma. These definitions tend to relate elder mistreatment to theories of caregiver stress [11].

A consensus conference of the National Center on Elder Abuse (NCEA) and the National Elder Abuse Incidence Study (NEAIS) has standardized definitions as follows [12]:

- **Physical abuse:** The use of physical force that might result in bodily injury, physical pain, or impairment. Physical punishments of any kind were examples of physical abuse.
- **Sexual abuse:** Nonconsensual sexual contact of any kind with an elderly person

- **Emotional or psychologic abuse:** The infliction of anguish, pain, or distress
- **Financial or material exploitation:** The illegal or improper use of an elder's funds, property, or assets
- **Abandonment:** The desertion of an elderly person by an individual who had physical custody or otherwise had assumed responsibility for providing care for an elder or by a person with physical custody of an elder
- **Neglect:** The refusal or failure to fulfill any part of a person, obligations, or duties to an elder
- **Self-neglect:** The behaviors of an elderly person that threaten his/her own health or safety. The definition of self neglect excludes a situation in which a mentally competent older person who understands the consequences of his/her decisions makes a conscious and voluntary decision to engage in acts that threaten his/her health or safety.

The standardization of these definitions is helpful for a variety of practical reasons and will likely have a positive effect on future study design. The area of self-neglect remains one of the greatest areas of variability among states.

Occurrence of elder abuse

It is believed that in the United States, over two million older adults are mistreated each year [13–15]. A landmark study by Pillemer and Finkelhor [14] revealed a prevalence rate of 32 per every 1000 adults. Physical abuse, verbal abuse, and neglect were found to be the most common types of mistreatment. Early studies found that 1% to 10% of seniors were victims of mistreatment [13,15]. All studies in this field acknowledge the ongoing belief that conceptual and methodologic flaws have led to our current underestimates [16,17]. Perhaps greater awareness of newer reporting guidelines will lead to increasingly improved estimates of the problem. There has been a 150% increase in reporting from 1986 to 1996 [18]. In 1996, the United States Administration on Aging study found that 551,011 persons over age 60 were victims of abuse, neglect, or self-neglect in a 1-year period [18]. In a study conducted in the Netherlands, four types of abuse (verbal aggression, physical aggression, financial mistreatment, and neglect) were studied in a cohort of community-dwelling residents aged 69 to 89. A prevalence rate of 56% was seen in this study group [19]. Limited data from Great Britain and Canada suggest similar trends [20,21]. A 4% incidence of abuse was noted in a small study completed in Maryland [22].

Risk factors for mistreatment include the following:

- Older age
- Lack of access to resources
- ow income
- Social isolation
- Minority status

- Low level of education
- Functional impairment
- Substance abuse by elder or caregiver
- Previous history of family violence
- History of psychologic problems
- Caregiver stress
- Cognitive impairment

Most studies show that women are more commonly victims than men. Pillemer's study is one exception [14]. Women often suffer physical abuse and are almost always the victims in sexual abuse. Men are more likely to live with others, whereas women are more likely to live alone, increasing their risk for self-neglect. A growing population of seniors will increase the risk for all types of elder mistreatment, including exploitation and abandonment [11,23–26].

Intuitively, it should follow that elder mistreatment is on the rise given a rapidly growing at risk population. This belief is reinforced by data showing the increasing number of reports made to protective services agencies [27–30]. The need to have accurate information at a national level is a compelling reason to have a standardized and required format by which states share information with a federal entity. It has been estimated that in 1988 there were 140,000 reports of elder abuse and that by 1996 that number had reached 293,000 [31]. An 11-year, longitudinal study by Lachs [32] was among the first to describe patterns in use of adult protective services agencies.

The United States Administration for Children and Families and the Administration on Aging conducted the NEAIS. The study was designed to identify reported and unreported cases of elder abuse and neglect in 1996 [33]. Understanding the gap between reported cases and unreported cases is critical. One of the goals of the NEAIS project was to collect incidence data that was generalizable to the entire country. Critics are concerned that this methodology will lead to significant underestimates that will not provide sufficiently compelling data needed to effect public policy [34]. Studies looking at the prevalence of elder mistreatment are less common but would likely reveal larger numbers if we had sound estimates of all existing cases of elder abuse.

Self-neglect as a form of abuse

Self-neglect is described as "the result of an adult's inability, due to physical or mental impairments or diminished capacity to perform essential self-care tasks including: providing essential food, clothing, shelter and medical care; obtaining goods and services necessary to maintain physical health, mental health, emotional well-being, and general safety; or managing financial affairs" by the National Association of Adult Protective Services Administrators [35]. Self-neglect presents one of greatest challenges in this field of study. Reports of self-neglect have increased 150% between 1986 and 1996 [24]. Data from regulatory agencies suggest that over 70% of reports they receive reflect self-neglect. People over age 80 may represent close to half of the cases of self-neglect [24].

Many of the risk factors for abuse and neglect are relevant to self-neglect. Functional dependence, alcohol or drug abuse, age, isolation, and psychiatric illness are accepted risk factors for self-neglect. A 1997 study by Lachs [32] found that cognitive impairment, poverty, and being of a nonwhite race were independent predictors for self-neglect. Lachs' 1998 [36] study revealed that self-neglect and mistreatment contribute to increased mortality rate. In his cohort, 73% of the protective services reports involved self-neglect. After a 13-year follow-up period, 40% of those in the self-neglect cohort (53.2% in the mistreatment cohort) had died during this period. Only 17% of the noninvestigated cohort died in the same period. In all three groups, cardiovascular events were the most common cause of death. Those experiencing self-neglect were more likely to end up in long-term care facilities. This was the first longitudinal study designed to look at the association between elder mistreatment and mortality.

Recognizing and understanding abusers

A better understanding of those who abuse is important for many reasons. By better identifying potential abusers, we may be able to intervene earlier or prevent mistreatment. Abusers are most often the primary caregiver. Adult children (50%) are more likely to abuse more than spouses (20% to 40%). Males abuse more than females. The abuser is often financially dependent on the victim [26,29]. Understanding the relationship between the abuser and the victim helps frame elder mistreatment in the continuum of domestic violence.

Theories of caregiver stress have been central to the attempts to better understand those who commit elder abuse. In a 1990 study by Homer and Gilleard [37], caregivers were studied over a 6-month period; 45% of the caregivers admitted to some type of abuse. Alcohol abuse was the most common risk factor for physical abuse. Previous abuse and a poor, long-standing relationship between caregiver and patient were other significant risk factors. In contrast to other studies, the degrees of mental and physical disability were not significantly associated with abuse [38].

Since the 1980s, we have appreciated the complexities of the relationship between abusers and their victims. It was learned that caregiver stress was not found to be a primary explanation for elder mistreatment. Despite the nuance in the studies of victims and abusers, few conclusions can be drawn to codify these complex relationships. Support for the caregiver stress theory remains in light of concerns that it is too one-dimensional to explain what is seen in practice or in research findings. Critics point out that this theory identifies the victim as the problem validates the abuser and may leave the victim in harm's way. Anetzberger's [39] explanatory model proposes that, primarily, characteristics of the perpetrator foster abuse; secondarily, characteristics of the victim, within a context, foster the abuse. She points out that caregiving is not the sole context. The model emphasizes the pathologies and perceptions of the perpetrator in her theoretical paradigm.

A 1989 study by Pillemer and Finkelhorn [40] provided additional support for caregiver personality issues as being important in the development of an abusive relationship. Their study compared theories of caregiver stress versus "problem relatives" (personality of the abusers). In this study, spouses—not adult children—were the larger group of offenders. Abuser deviance and dependence (and life stress in nonspouse caregivers) were far more important predictors of mistreatment by caregivers than were characteristics of the victims (eg, level of disability). This further serves to place elder mistreatment in the traditional realm of domestic violence while repositioning the important topic of caregiver stress in the menu of issues important to geriatric care.

Ramsey-Klawsnik [41] proposes the following five types of offenders. This theoretical construct is based on experience in forensic investigations and clinical evaluations and treatment to victims and perpetrators of elder mistreatment.

- **The overwhelmed:** This group is well intentioned and generally qualified to provide care. When care needs exceed what they can provide, they may abuse verbally or physically. They do not look for victims.
- **The impaired:** This group is well intentioned but has problems that prevent them from delivering care. These caregivers may suffer from mental or physical problems that serve as barriers to providing adequate care. They may be unaware of the deficits in their care delivery. Neglect is more common in this group, and they may tend to control the victim through abuse.
- **The narcissistic:** These caregivers enter into caregiving relationships to meet their own needs. They are more likely to steal from seniors and neglect them. They see the relationship as a means to an end and may be attracted to nursing homes or centers where they can enter into relationships with vulnerable adults.
- **The domineering or bullying:** This group may feel entitled to exert power and authority. They may have narcissistic tendencies and often feel that the victim deserved the maltreatment. This type of offender may honor limits in other settings and has insight into the nature of the maladaptive behavior. This type of offender is prone to neglect and financial abuse. This type of offender may engage in sexual abuse.
- **The sadistic:** Offenders of this type often have sociopathic personalities and take pleasure in the mistreatment of their victim. Their abuse of others allows them to have feelings of power and importance.

These personality profiles may be helpful in research and clinical settings. This information has special significance for those responsible for hiring workers in long-term care facilities and other institutions.

Identifying elder abuse

The reporting of elder abuse remains a central concern in responding to elder abuse and neglect. Elder mistreatment is under-reported. For example, in Illinois there were 76,000 victims over age 60, but only 8000 reports were made [41]. All states have reporting mechanisms in place [42]. Much has been done to aggregate data at the national level. Tatara [29] pointed out the significant differences in definitions and eligibility among states. She estimated that there were 140,000 reports in 1988, which represented a 19.7% increase form 1986. Data from the NCEA revealed a reporting incidence of 293,000 by 1996. In 1991, the National Aging Resource Center on Elder Abuse surveyed the 54 jurisdictions and asked 12 basic questions regarding the agencies' local data. It represented the first study of this scope. Although many of the questions had low response rates, a great deal was learned about incidence, characteristics of abusers, victims, type of abuse, substantiation of reports, and self-neglect.

Wolf and Li [30] studied factors in reporting elder abuse within 27 geographic areas in Massachusetts in 1994. Four of 10 factors were found to be significant: lower socioeconomic status of the older adult, more community training of area professionals, higher agency service rating scores, and a lower community agency-protective services relationship score were predictors of higher reporting rates.

The AMA's Diagnostic and Treatment Guidelines on Elder Abuse and Neglect represent a starting point for physicians to learn about their role in the recognition and response to mistreatment [9]. Despite being well positioned to report elder abuse, physicians report infrequently [43–47]. Despite reporter fear of being wrong, the majority of reports are substantiated. One large survey suggests that reporters are home care workers (27%), physicians and other health care professionals (18%), and family members (15%) [29]. A review of 5 years of elder abuse reports in Michigan found that physicians made only 2% of the reports; community members (41%), nonphysician health care providers (26%), social and mental health workers (25%), and law enforcement officials (5%) were more likely to report [48].

A 1997 survey of emergency medicine physicians revealed that of 705 respondents, only 31% were aware of a written protocol for reporting elder abuse, and they were largely unfamiliar with their state law. Unclear definitions, the inability to identify abuse and neglect, and concerns about resources were the common concerns raised in this study. Only 25% received instruction on the topic in residency training. Other common concerns raised by physicians include fear of being incorrect and disturbing the doctor-patient relationship [44].

Educating and encouraging physicians and other clinicians to learn to discuss the topic of domestic violence in late life can be helpful. Box 1 provides questions that can serve as a starting point for conversations with patients. These discussions should be private, and the alleged abuser should not be present during the initial conversation.

Physical examination of the older adult may not always provide clear evidence of abuse or neglect. Fulmer and Ashley [16] attempted to clarify the clinical

---

Box 1. Elder abuse screening questions

- Has anyone at home hurt you?
- Has anyone ever touched you without your consent?
- Has anyone ever made you do things you didn't want to do?
- Has anyone taken anything that was yours without asking?
- Has anyone ever scolded or threatened you?
- Have you ever signed any documents that you didn't understand?
- Are you afraid of anyone at home?
- Are you alone a lot?
- Has anyone ever failed to help you take care of yourself when you needed help?

Adapted from Elder mistreatment guidelines for health care professionals: detection, assessment and intervention, Mount Sinai/Victim Services Agency Elder Abuse Project. New York: 1988; with permission.

---

indicators of neglect. In their Elder Assessment Instrument, they included nine indicators: poor hygiene, poor nutrition, poor skin integrity, contractures, excoriations, pressure ulcers, dehydration, impaction, and malnutrition. Despite limits to this 1989 study, many of these items are important quality indicators for regulatory agencies that oversee hospitals and long-term care facilities. Box 2 summarizes potential findings that may suggest abuse or neglect.

Elder abuse in special populations

There may be significant barriers in using the examination in patients with late-stage disease. The natural history of advanced neurologic disease (eg, Alzheimer disease [AD], Parkinson disease, and amyotrophic lateral sclerosis), cancer, or end-stage cardiopulmonary disease may lead to severe debility. Individuals who are immobile are at risk for many problems, such pressure ulcers, pneumonia, and venous thromboembolism. Therefore, it is sometimes difficult to know what would have been preventable with adequate care. These issues are of particular importance for nursing home residents and nonverbal adults. Defining neglect against the backdrop of severe, chronic illness can challenge the most sophisticated clinician. Dementia and long-term care facilities have complex relationships with elder mistreatment and are addressed in detail elsewhere in this issue. Depression and dementia are common in long-term care facilities. Depression and dementia may be prevalent in elder mistreatment [40,49,50].

Box 2. Physical indicators of elder abuse

Physical abuse

    Bruises, wound, burns: unexplained, of various ages, patterns,
        well-defined shapes, immersion pattern
    Rope or restraint marks on wrists or ankles
    Traumatic alopecia or scalp swelling

Psychologic abuse

    Habit disorder (sucking, rocking)
    Neurotic disorders
    Conduct disorder

Sexual abuse

    Genital or anal pain, itching, bruising, or bleeding
    Venereal disease
    Torn, stained, or bloody underwear

Neglect

    Dehydration, malnutrition
    Poor hygiene
    Inappropriate dress
    Unattended physical or medical needs
    Extensive pressure ulcers
    Excoriations
    Fecal impaction

    Long-term care facilities have been a central focus of concern with regard to elder mistreatment since the 1960s. Concerns of the privation of residents' rights and substandard care have prevailed since that time. Anecdotes has often prevailed because there have been formidable barriers to research of any kind in this setting. In 1973, Kahana [51] wrote: "Those few accounts which look at the quality of life in institutions for the aged at close range tend to conjure up images of Dante's *Inferno* . . . . . . Nevertheless, there are no hard data on the prevalence of inhumane treatment in various institutional settings. Consequently there is the possibility that we are interpreting the isolated or occasional event as the norm." It is recognized that nursing home residents are increasingly dependent (Table 1). It is not uncommon that nursing home residents may be

Table 1
Characteristics of nursing home residents

Characteristics	Percent
Aged ≥85 yr	49
Nonwhite	9
Receives assistance with ≥3 ADLs	83
Mild to moderate cognitive impairment	71
Exhibits physically aggressive behaviors	9
Exhibits any behaviors (eg, verbally or physically aggressive, resists nursing care, socially inappropriate)	30

Abbreviation: ADL, activities of daily living.
Data from Krauss NA, Altman BM. Characteristics of nursing home residents-1996 (AHCPR pub No. 99-0006). Rockville, MD: Agency for Health Care Policy and Research. MEPS Research Findings No. 5.1998.

"unbefriended elders." A population of elders without meaningful advocates is growing [52].

Since the 1960s, qualitative studies describing mistreatment in nursing homes appeared in journals as case reports. It was difficult to know whether these were observations of isolated incidents or significant trends. A 1984 article by Monk [53] analyzed federal and state data and revealed that these were underestimates. A 1989 study by Pillemer and Moore [40] presented data from a random sample of 577 nurses and nursing aides from long-term care facilities. Self-report from staff showed psychologic, physical, and verbal abuse was not uncommon. Thirty-six percent of respondents had witnessed at least one act of physical abuse in the previous year.

A GAO report suggests that 50% of reports of physical or sexual abuse in nursing homes are not received until 2 or more days after the incident has been discovered. GAO data underscore the observation that the penalties for abuse in these institutions are often mild [54]. The need to develop reliable programs to screen potential nursing home employees remains a pressing issue.

Employees working for low wages in a stressful environment who are the hands-on caregivers are likely at high risk to become abusers. Twenty years after the initial studies, many of the issues remain the same with regard to the work-force and the environment in long-term care facilities despite dramatic increases in regulatory oversight. These ongoing circumstances compel us to develop staff education programs that are intended to decrease mistreatment [55].

The special relationship that exists among dementia, elder mistreatment, and nursing home care are discussed in detail elsewhere in this issue. The prevalence of AD increases with age, and AD will affect 14 million Americans by the year 2040. Despite conflicting data, it is often thought to be a risk factor for abuse and neglect. The functional decline marked by cognitive and physical decrements eventually results in decisional incapacity and the need for 24-hour care and surrogate decision makers [56]. In the community setting, AD has been identified as a risk factor for family violence. A study of 184 community-dwelling patients with AD and their caregivers found that 5.4% of caregivers were violent toward the patient and that there was 17.4% prevalence of violence. Aggressive behavior may be seen in 57% to 67% of patients with dementia [57].

Advanced AD is a common cause for nursing home placement. This population is particularly vulnerable because of the degree of dependency and associated behavioral problems. Falls, agitation, dehydration, malnutrition, and worsening physical health may be indicators of abuse and neglect. The natural course of AD and other primary progressive dementias often makes such declines difficult to interpret as to whether or not the status change is expected. The growing population of nursing home residents with dementia challenges a system that is already flawed and filled with risk factors for mistreatment.

There is a growing awareness that the causes of death of nursing home residents are often unknown. Deaths of individuals with long-standing, chronic illness with multiple comorbidities often go uninvestigated. A study of 2400 deaths in Arkansas nursing homes found 50 cases of suspected abuse or neglect. There is increasing recognition that there may be a much larger role for forensic studies in the unexplained deaths of older adults from long-term care centers and from the community [58].

Innovative examples in nontraditional nursing home care offer promise with regard to the prevention of elder abuse in the long-term care setting. The Pioneer Network model is intended to form collaborative partnerships among stakeholders in long-term care: residents, families, resident advocates, staff, and surveyors. This management style is intended to promote well-being for staff through mentorship and relationship building [59]. The Coalition for the Rights of the Infirm Elderly has developed training methods for nursing home personnel to prevent abusive behavior. Limited data have revealed less abuse and burnout and fewer conflictual interactions with residents [55]. The Wellspring Model for Improving Nursing Home Quality has demonstrated enhancement of care and relationship through education and support of front-line staff [60].

Future implications for the health care team

The core philosophy of geriatric medicine is reflected in an ongoing commitment to interdisciplinary care. The effectiveness of team care has been shown in a variety of settings. As suggested by Lachs [46], if we begin to think of elder abuse and neglect as a geriatric syndrome, it follows that the same analytic and collaborative approach will be helpful. Screening tools need to be developed for identifying domestic violence in later life in the same way we have developed tools for many of the other geriatric syndromes. These basic principles are easily taught to students in all disciplines.

Frail, older adults with complex needs rely not only on the contributions of a variety of health care professionals but also on new team members that may include representatives from the legal, financial, and protective service communities [61,62]. Dyer's model program [63] was created to treat elder neglect. It represents an effective and successful example of collaboration between a geriatrics team and APS workers by incorporating essential elements of geriatric assessment in the evaluation of neglect. They demonstrated that isolated seniors might be more agreeable to comprehensive geriatric assessment than to traditional psychiatric evaluation. This has great implications for the growing population of unbefriended elders with questionable decisional capacity. Dyer identified the need for culturally sensitive approaches to the evaluation of neglect.

Geriatricians are appropriate leaders in the evaluation of potential abuse and neglect victims because they are trained in the interface of medical and psychiatric issues and are vigilant in recognizing and analyzing syndromes that lead to functional decline in the broadest sense. They are also sensitized to clinical findings that may suggest mistreatment. Comprehensive geriatric assessment is often appropriate for older adults who are being investigated for mistreatment because the medical piece of the evaluation is often missing from the traditional evaluation [64,65]. The utility of an expanded concept of the geriatric assessment team holds great promise. It is essential that we succeed in getting more people to join the team. "Abuse may go undetected until observant professionals intervene" [66].

References

[1] The Program Resources Department, The American Association of Retired Persons, and the Administration on Aging. A profile of older Americans. Washington, DC: US Department of Health and Human Services; 1993.
[2] Elder abuse: an assessment of the federal response. Washington, DC: Select Committee on Aging House of Representatives, Subcommittee on Human Services; 1989.
[3] de Beauvoir S. Old age. London: Penguin Group; 1977.
[4] Shakespeare W. King Lear. Act 2, scene 3.
[5] Swift J. Gulliver's Travels. Part III, chapter X. Penguin Books Ltd., 1960.
[6] Burston GR. Granny battering. BMJ 1975;3:592.
[7] US House Select Committee on Aging and US House Science and Technology Subcommittee on Domestic, International, Scientific Planning, Analysis and Cooperation. Domestic violence. Washington, DC: US Government Printing Office; 1978.
[8] Subcommittee on Health and Long-Term Care of the Select Committee on Aging House of Representatives. Elder abuse: a decade of shame and inaction. Washington, DC: US Government Printing Office; 1990.
[9] AMA Council on Judicial and Ethical Affairs. Physicians and domestic violence: ethical considerations. JAMA 1992;267:113–6.
[10] US House of Representatives HR1674 The Elder Abuse Prevention, Identification, and Treatment Act. 1985.
[11] O'Malley TA, O'Malley HC, Everitt DE, et al. Categories of family-mediated abuse and neglect of elderly persons. J Am Geriatr Soc 1984;32:362–9.
[12] Tatara T. Suggested state guidelines for gathering and reporting domestic elder abuse statistics for compiling national data. Washington, DC: National Aging Resource Center on Elder Abuse; 1990.
[13] Gioglio GR, Blakemore P. Elder abuse in New Jersey: the knowledge and experience of abuse among older New Jerseyans. Trenton (NJ): Department of Human Services; 1983.
[14] Pillemer K, Finkelhor D. The prevalence of elder abuse: a random sample survey. Gerontologist 1988;28:51–7.

[15] Tatara T. Elder abuse in the United States: an issue paper. Washington, DC: National Aging Resource Center on Elder Abuse; 1990.

[16] Fulmer T, Ashley J. Clinical indicators of elder neglect. Appl Nurs Res 1989;2:161–7.

[17] Wolf RS. Elder abuse: ten years later. J Am Geriatr Soc 1988;36:758–62.

[18] National Center on Elder Abuse. National elder abuse incident final report. Washington DC: Administration for Children and Families, Administration on Aging, US Department on Health and Human Services; 1998.

[19] Comijs HC, Pot AM, Smit JH, et al. Elder abuse in the community: prevalence and consequences. J Am Geriatr Soc 1998;46:885–8.

[20] Ogg J, Bennett G. Elder abuse in Britain. BMJ 1992;305:988–9.

[21] Podnieks E. National survey on abuse of the elderly in Canada. J Elder Abuse Negl 1992;4:5–58.

[22] Block MR, Sinnott JD. The battered elder syndrome: an exploratory study. College Park (MD): Center on Aging; 1979.

[23] Comijs HC, Smit JH, Pot AM, et al. Risk indicators of elder mistreatment in the community. J Elder Abuse Negl 1998;9:67–76.

[24] Lachs MS, Pillmer K. Abuse and neglect of elderly persons. New Engl J Med 1995;332:437–43.

[25] Lachs MS, Williams C, O'Brien S, et al. Risk factors for reported elder abuse and neglect: a nine-year observational cohort study. Gerontologist 1997;37:469–74.

[26] Pillemer K, Suitor JJ. Violence and violent feelings: what causes them among family caregivers? J Gerontol 1992;47:S165–72.

[27] Bird PE, Harrington DT, Barillo DJ, et al. Elder abuse: a call to action. J Burn Care Rehabil 1998;19:522–7.

[28] Pavlik VN, Hyman DJ, Festa NA, et al. Quantifying the problem of abuse and neglect in adults: analysis of a statewide database. J Am Geriatr Soc 2001;49:45–8.

[29] Tatara T. Understanding the nature and scope of domestic elder abuse with the use of state aggregate date: summaries of the key findings of a national survey of state APS and aging agencies. J Elder Abuse Negl 1993;5:35–57.

[30] Wolf RS, Li D. Factors affecting the rate of elder abuse reporting to a state protective services program. Gerontologist 1999;39:222–8.

[31] Tatara T. Summaries of national elder abuse data: an exploratory study of state statistics based on a survey of state adult protective service and aging agencies. Washington, DC: National Aging Resource Center on Elder Abuse; 1990.

[32] Lachs MS, Williams C, O'Brien S, et al. Older adults: an 11-year longitudinal study of adult protective service use. Arch Intern Med 1996;156:449–53.

[33] Thomas C. The first national study of elder abuse and neglect: contrast with results from other studies. J Elder Abuse Negl 2000;12:1–14.

[34] Quinn KM. Testimony submitted to the Senate Subcommittee on Aging. Washington, DC: National Association of Adult Protective Services Administrators; 1999.

[35] Rathbone-McCuan E, Fabian DR. Self-neglecting elders: a clinical dilemma. New York: Auburn House; 1992.

[36] Lachs MS, Williams CS, O'Brien S, et al. The mortality of elder mistreatment. JAMA 1998; 280:428–32.

[37] Homer AC, Gilleard C. Abuse of elderly people by their carers. BMJ 1990;301:1359–62.

[38] Fulmer T, Anetzberger GJ. Knowledge about family violence interventions in the field of elder abuse. Washington, DC: Committee on the Assessment of Family Violence Interventions of the National Research Council and Institute of Medicine; 1995.

[39] Anetzberger GJ. Caregiving: primary cause of elder abuse? Generations 2000;2:46–51.

[40] Pillemer K, Moore DW. Abuse of patients in nursing homes: findings from a survey of staff. Gerontologist 1989;29:314–20.

[41] Ramsey-Klawsnik H. Elder-abuse offenders: a typology. Generations 2000;2:17–22.

[42] Bonnie RJ, Wallace RB, editors. Elder mistreatment: abuse, neglect, and exploitation in an aging America. Washington, DC: The National Academies Press; 2003. p. 181–237.

[43] Jones J, Doughherty J, Schelble D, et al. Emergency department protocol for the diagnosis and evaluation of geriatric abuse. Ann Emerg Med 1988;17:1006–15.

[44] Jones JS, Veenstra TR, Seamon JP, et al. Elder mistreatment: national survey of emergency physicians. Ann Emerg Med 1997;30:473–9.

[45] Kleinschmidt KC. Elder abuse: a review. Ann Emerg Med 1997;30:463–72.

[46] Lachs MS. Preaching to the unconverted: educating physicians about elder abuse. J Elder Abuse Negl 1995;7:1–12.

[47] Senn DR, McDowell JD, Alder ME. Dentistry's role in the recognition and reporting of domestic violence, abuse, and neglect. Dent Clin North Am 2001;45:343–63.

[48] Rosenblatt DE, Cho KH, Durance PW. Reporting mistreatment of older adults: the rold of physicians. J Am Geriatr Soc 1996;44:65–70.

[49] Dyer CB, Pavlik VN, Murphy KP, et al. The high prevalence of depression and dementia in elder abuse or neglect. J Am Geriatr Soc 2000;48:205–8.

[50] Stannard C. Old folks and dirty work: the social conditions for patient abuse in a nursing home. Soc Probl 1973;20:329–42.

[51] Kahana E. The humane treatment of old people in institutions. Gerontologist 1973;13:282–8.

[52] Karp N, Wood E. Incapacitated and alone: health care decision-making for the unbefriended elderly. Washington (DC): American Bar Association Commission on Law and Aging; 2003.

[53] Monk A, Kaye LW, Litwin H. Resolving grievances in the nursing home: a study of the ombudsman program. New York: Columbia University Press; 1974.

[54] Nursing homes: more can be done to protect residents from abuse. Washington, DC: United States General Accounting Office; 2002.

[55] Menio D, Keller BH. CARIE: a multifaceted approach to abuse prevention in nursing homes. Generations 2000;2:28–32.

[56] Reuben DB, Yoshikawa TT, Besdine RW, editors. Geriatrics review syllabus: a core curriculum in geriatric medicine. 3rd edition. Dubuque (IA): Kendall/Hunt Publishing Company; 1996. p. 107–10.

[57] Paveza GJ, Cohen D, Eisdorfer C, et al. Severe family violence and Alzheimer's disease: prevalence and risk factors. Gerontologist 1992;32:493–7.

[58] Ortmann C, Fechner G, Bajanowski T, et al. Fatal neglect of the elderly. Int J Legal Med 2001;114:191–3.

[59] The pioneer challenge-changing the culture of long-term care. Available at: www.asaging.org/at/at-212/pioneers.html. Accessed October 8, 2002.

[60] Stone RI, Reinhard C, Bowers B, et al. Evaluation of the Wellspring Model for Improving Nursing Home Quality. Washington, DC: The Commonwealth Fund; 2003.

[61] Davis GG, Carroll JL, Barber D, et al. Investigation of long-term care deaths within a medical examiner system. Ann Long-Term Care 2003;11:29–32.

[62] Hodge PD. National law enforcement programs to prevent, detect, investigate, and prosecute elder abuse and neglect in health care facilities. J Elder Abuse Negl 1998;9:23–39.

[63] Dyer CB, Gleason MS, Murphy KP, et al. Treating elder neglect: collaboration between a geriatrics assessment team and adult protective services. South Med J 1999;92:242–4.

[64] Dyer CB, Goins AM. The role of interdisciplinary geriatric assessment in addressing self-neglect of the elderly. Generations 2000;2:23–7.

[65] Harrell R, Toronjo CH, Mclaughlin J. How geriatricians identify elder abuse and neglect. Am J Med Sci 2002;323:34–8.

[66] Turkoski BB. Ethical dilemma: is this elder abuse? Home Healthc Nurse 2003;21:518–21.

ELSEVIER
SAUNDERS

Clin Geriatr Med 21 (2005) 293–313

CLINICS IN
GERIATRIC
MEDICINE

Medical Implications of Elder Abuse and Neglect

XinQi Dong, MD

*Section of Geriatrics, Department of Medicine, University of Chicago, 5841 South Maryland Avenue,
MC 6098, Chicago, IL 60637, USA*

Health care professionals' recognition of elder abuse and neglect as a problem is a relatively recent phenomenon; its appearance in the medical literature began within the last 30 years. An estimated 2 million American elderly persons experience abuse and neglect each year, and most of them experience abuse repeatedly and in multiple forms [1]. Estimates on the incidence and prevalence of abuse and neglect of persons 60 years of age and older have ranged from 3 to 40 per 1000 to as high as 100 to 120 per 1000, depending on the definition used and population studied [2–5].

Despite the accessibility of adult protective services and nursing home regulations in all 50 states and mandatory reporting laws for elder abuse and neglect in most states, an overwhelming number of abused and neglected elderly persons pass through our health care system undetected and untreated [6,7]. Many cases involve subtle signs, such as poor hygiene or dehydration, and can easily be missed. It is estimated that only 1 in 14 cases of elder abuse and neglect comes to the attention of authorities [8,9]. The medical implications of elder abuse and neglect can be devastating [10]. The quality of life can be jeopardized in the forms of declining functional abilities, progressive dependency, a sense of helplessness, social isolation, and a cycle of worsening stress and psychologic decline. The health implications of abuse and neglect include its associations with premature mortality and morbidity [11–14]. It can induce fractures, depression, dementia, malnutrition, and death [14–16]. It was found that the risk of death for elder abuse and neglect victims are three times higher than for nonvictims [17]. The direct medical costs associated with these violent injuries are estimated to add over $5.3 billion to the nation's annual health expenditures [18].

E-mail address: xdong@medicine.bsd.uchicago.edu

0749-0690/05/$ – see front matter © 2005 Elsevier Inc. All rights reserved.
doi:10.1016/j.cger.2004.10.006
geriatric.theclinics.com

Over the last few decades, the child abuse movement has prompted extensive investigation and publicity, but attention to elder abuse and neglect has been relatively lacking in the medical and legal arenas. The notion of "granny-battering" was initially introduced as a letter to the editor in the British Medical Journal in 1975 that contained multiple descriptions of elder abuse and neglect perpetrated by family members [19]. Since that time, physicians have endeavored to define and raise awareness of the prevalence of elder abuse and neglect.

Despite the relatively recent increase in awareness of elder abuse and neglect, physicians report only 2% of all elder abuse and neglect cases [20,21]. There are many barriers for physicians and other health care professionals to report suspected cases of elder abuse and neglect. Health care professionals often are unaware of state laws or disregard them [22,23]. They are concerned about angering the abusers, possible court appearances, and possible damage to professional relationships with clients. They feel skeptical about investigative follow-up, lack confidence in support services, doubt the ability to recognize abuse, lack cooperation by clients or families, and lack time and reimbursement for time spent, and they ear involvement [24]. Through education, training, and reinforcement at local, state, and national levels, health care professionals can be more involved, raise suspicions, and be advocates for the vulnerable victims of abuse and neglect.

Quality of life

Functional decline and dependency

Functional status is the foundation of geriatric medicine and has a direct impact on an elder's ability to live successfully within their environment [25]. Compromised functional status is also a logical consequence of abuse and neglect regardless of whether the immediate impact of mistreatment is physical, psychologic, or both. Physical health, mental health, and functional ability are distinct but often inseparable factors in the aging elderly population. Older people who have difficulty performing activities of daily living (ADLs) are more often neglected, particularly if their problem involves eating [26,27]. Demented patients who cannot perform ADLs sustain more physical abuse [28]. Neglect most commonly affects those who have no one to turn to for help, are in poor health, are poorly functioning, or live alone [29]. This creates a cycle of progressive inability to form daily functions as the result of mistreatment and increases the risk for additional insults of abuse and neglect.

Other studies have suggested that functional impairment leads to dependency and vulnerability in elderly persons [30,31]. Most people understand that older adults may need some assistance, but being primarily dependent on others over prolonged periods of time is looked upon negatively by older people themselves or by those who must care for them. Such dependency is often viewed with fear, dread, disrespect, embarrassment, and disapproval. We accept dependency in children because we understand that children need their parents for survival, but children grow up and gradually become less dependent. This is not true for elderly persons who become functionally dependent because of physical or mental impairments. These impairments are likely to deteriorate over time given the nature of chronic illness. The older adult becomes gradually more dependent and therefore more defenseless to the action of abuse and neglect [32]. The type of dependencies encountered can include economic dependency as the individual moves from being a producer to a consumer; physical dependency arising from waning physical strength and energy and diminishing ability to perform ADLs; social dependency accruing if mobility becomes problematic; and emotional dependency, often a corollary of the other forms of dependency [33].

Self-rated health and helplessness

Poor self-reported health is strongly associated with mortality and adverse health outcomes, and good self-reported health is generally correlated with well-being [34,35]. Elderly persons who are abused and neglected suffer many losses and progressive declining health status. From the Missing Voices Series, elderly persons in eight countries were surveyed regarding the effect of abuse and neglect [36]. The subjects expressed desperation on the feeling of insecurity, loss of dignity, disrespect, and poor state of health as a result of abuse and neglect. The vulnerable elderly persons often stated, "one rude word said to an old man is stronger than stabbing him with a knife" and "respect is better than food and drink." Given the expansion and modernization of many developing countries, many elderly persons from this series felt that family bonds are collapsing, in so much as there is less respect and more carelessness toward elders, and that their health is suffering as a result of such mistreatment.

Frequently, the older person reacts to abuse and neglect with denial, resignation, withdrawal, fear, or depression. These reactions can result in feelings of guilt, shame, helplessness, and worthlessness. Through the multiple losses of power that can come with old age, some elders may feel that they are a burden to others. Some older people react by becoming more submissive, which may invite more abuse and neglect by a malicious or unsympathetic caregiver. Many older people believe that events are beyond their control, and feelings of impotence take root. The elder, helpless to change the abusive environment, stops trying to do anything and accepts whatever treatment is presented. This phenomenon was described by Seligman [37], who termed it "learned helplessness." Seligman postulated that helplessness produces emotional disturbances. The motivation to respond to a situation is exhausted if the elderly person feels that nothing can be done to affect the outcome. This is also due to an increased inability to perceive success. The elder may do something that changes the situation for the better but may not be aware of the success or may not fully realize that his or her action had made a difference. Hence, even success becomes failure. Such perceived helplessness produces fear as long as the person is uncertain of being able to influence what happens, and then it produces depression.

Fear and social isolation

Access to the abused and neglected elderly person can be difficult for the health care providers because the perpetrator may block the efforts to intervene and further induce isolation of the victim. As a reaction to the abuse and neglect, most victims react with anger, disappointment, fear, or grief. At other times, the elderly patient does not cooperate with the health care worker who provides services to take action toward the alleged abuser because they believe that little can be done to improve their situation and fear further mistreatment [38]. If elderly people perceive investigation of abuse and neglect as an intrusion into their lives, they demonstrate this through resistance to the service provided [39]. Resistance may be demonstrated by the elderly clients directly or indirectly, letting the elder abuse investigator know that they are uncomfortable with the service provided and that their discomfort will be reflected in the outcome of the service process. That is, there will be lower rates of substantiation, higher rates of service refusal, and a gap between service needed and that provided.

Lau and Kosberg [40] found that many elderly persons judged to have been abused and neglected often denied the existence of any problem and became progressively isolated. Among a multitude of explanations are fear of retaliation, embarrassment, unwillingness to initiate legal action, trepidation that the solution to the problem will be worse than the problem itself, beliefs that they are being "paid back" for their earlier abusive behaviors, and perceiving their dependence as the cause of the problem. Many older people are concerned about their family privacy and fear public exposure and the embarrassment and humiliation that such exposure brings. They may worry that they will not be believed because the alleged abuser may act differently in public. A study of black, white, and Korean American subjects showed differences in perception of abuse and neglect and in help-seeking patterns [41]. The study identified differences in formal and informal help-seeking attitudes between groups. Korean Americans were much more tolerant of abusive situations and less likely to seek help, which further induced social isolation. They did not want to reveal "family shame" to others or create conflict among their relatives, yet they were not able to any external help in their environment and alleviate the causes of the abuse and neglect. When the alleged abuser is an adult child, the victim may feel disgraced for having raised a child who would betray him or her in any way.

Elderly persons and their caregivers are often caught together in emotional turmoil that they often cannot comprehend and for which there are no easy solutions. There are circumstances in the lives of older persons that make the caregiver role difficult to maintain. Older persons tend to lose their roles, suffer losses that cannot be recovered, and require more services than what are available to them. Linked to these feelings of shame and embarrassment is anxiety about what will happen when others find out about the abuse and neglect. They do not want to admit their vulnerabilities, betray loved ones, or report abuse and neglect to the authorities or outsiders. Victims of abuse and neglect may fear that losing a caregiver will result in institutionalization. Their fear may be true, as reflected in a Connecticut study in which 60% of abused and neglected victims admitted for short-term care remained institutionalized permanently [42]. The older person may realistically fear that if the abuse and neglect is reported, the perpetrator will strike back with additional mistreatment. Alleged abusers may threaten to inflict more severe abuse, destroy property or pets, or even kill their victims, other loved ones, or themselves [43].

Stress and psychologic decline

Over the last few decades of research, stress and stress life events have been linked to the onset of illness and other maladaptive behavior at the individual and societal levels. There are many harmful physical and psychologic consequences of stress (eg, the development of coronary disease) [44–46]. Stress-induced psychologic decline in the life of the patient is strongly correlated with drug noncompliance [47]. Stress has also been associated with the development of aggression directed inward in the form of suicide and outward in the form of violent behaviors [48]. Victims of abuse and neglect suffer more than just the debilitating physical or material consequences of the acts. Becoming a victim challenges most people's basic assumptions about safety and security. Research has demonstrated that victims of crime begin to question themselves and begin to see themselves as weak, frightened, out of control, powerless, and lacking a sense of autonomy [49].

Psychologic abuse of elderly persons is generally seen as the blatant, subtle, or demeaning verbal rejection of an elderly person who subsequently experiences psychologic stress or trauma. This is frequently observed in the caregiver of an elderly parent when the family feels hopelessly confined by the needs of the elderly person. They often express themselves as verbalized desires to return to the lives they previously enjoyed [50]. It has been well documented that negative interpersonal interactions strongly predict a variety of negative psychologic outcomes and are strongly related to distress [51–53].

Dyer et al [16], in a case-controlled study of elderly patients referred for abuse and neglect to a geriatric assessment clinic, found a higher prevalence of depression in victims of mistreatment compared with patients referred for other reasons. When depression is obvious, it can include feelings of helplessness and hopelessness, a frequent sense of guilt, loneliness, despair, fear of death, loss of interest in sex, and loss of appetite. Victims of elder abuse and neglect tend to blame themselves for the abuse and harbor much guilt and low self-esteem [29].

Other studies have highlighted the individual's relative ignorance of psychologic abuse in contrast to physical abuse, perhaps in part because of the difficulty in identifying observable consequences of the victim of psychologic abuse [54]. Neville et al [55] found that the most common reasons for psychiatric admission for such a population were behavior problems, self-neglect, psychotic symptoms, and other psychiatric illness. Sensitivity to the psychologic states of elder abuse and neglect may be especially important because it may assist in the early and accurate identification of elderly persons at risk. Such elderly persons may be more prone to depression and may engage in suicide and other methods of self-destructive behavior [56,57].

Morbidity and mortality

Health care system use

Elder abuse and neglect are recently recognized forms of family violence, but much less is known compared with child or spousal abuse. Little is known about how patients of elder abuse and neglect interact with the health care system. The victims of elder abuse and neglect are more likely to have multiple complaints and frequent presentations in ambulatory care setting. Mouton and Espino [58] found that older women who experienced abuse were likely to consult medical practitioners with conditions such as physical injuries, gynecologic complaints, gastrointestinal disorders, fatigue, headache, myalgias, depression, and anxiety. It is estimated that worldwide 10% to 50% of women reported have been physically assaulted at some point in their adult lives and that 14% to 25% of women seen at ambulatory medical clinics and 20% of women seen in emergency departments (EDs) have been physically abused [12,13]. In outpatient medical practice, symptoms of these presentations are often treated, but the true underlying abuse and neglect of the elderly are left to be discovered. Those patients often have nonspecific presentations to the outpatient settings. An effective strategy to address family violence in all its forms in the non-emergent outpatient setting would improve the quality of life for those individuals and perhaps would reduce health care cost.

Older patients use emergency medical services at twice the rate of other age groups [59,60] and represent 22% of emergency medical service users in one urban study [61]. The geriatric population is the fastest growing age group in the United States, comprising 13% of the population in 1990 and possibly 18% in 2020 and 25% in 2050 [24,62]. The population of people over age 85 will more than double during the same time. With the simultaneous decline in the pediatric population, the elderly will outnumber children by the year 2020 [27,63]. Most likely, ED physicians will treat an increasing number of geriatric patients for illness, injury, abuse, and neglect.

A study of urban emergency room (ER) uses found that abused and neglected community elders recognized through a state elderly protective services program are more likely to come to the ER for assessment and treatment [64]. One fourth of ER visits had ICD-9 codes consistent with injury, and 66% of the subjects who used emergency services had at least one ER visit with injury-related discharge diagnosis or chief complaint. No single injury type or chief complaint emerged as highly prevalent in this population. Jones et al [65] retrospectively examined medical records of elder abuse and neglect cases that were identified through the ER. In this study, elder neglect presented to the ER exceeded physical abuse, bruises, lacerations, and other injuries. Other presentations of abuse and neglect included dehydration, fractures, and failure to thrive.

The metaphor of a "frequent flyer" in the ER should raise caution to health care professionals, especially relating to the magnitude of an elderly patient's health care needs. Becoming aware of those repeated presentations to the ER should lead us to explore in greater detail the nature of the elder's health status and medical management and to express concern about the adequacy of the elder's health care management by caregivers and health care professionals. We should consider our elderly patients who have recurrent visits to the ER to be at greater risk for abuse and neglect [66]. The high flow of a busy ER should not be seen as an impediment for care but as an opportunity to influence the lives of frail elderly persons.

Hospitalization is one of the most costly health care system interventions. Often, the severely abused and neglected elderly person requires hospitalization. In one study, more than 30% of ER visits by abused and neglected elders resulted in hospital admission [64]. They often present with dehydration, fracture, failure to thrive, or need of long-term placement, but this intervention is not necessarily being perceived as a dire outcome. It may give the health care professionals a chance to be able to take the victims out of the abusive and neglectful environment to have a chance to inquire about possible abuse and neglect and to reverse the physical and medical consequences of such mistreatment. The ER use and hospital admission in the abused and neglected population may also have higher cost to the health care system. Although there are no rigorous scientific data documenting true cost of elder abuse and neglect, it is suspected to be high.

Nursing home placement

Adult Protective Services is the official state entity charged with promoting advocacy and protecting victims of elder abuse and neglect. Elderly persons referred to protective services represent some of the most frail, isolated, and medically and psychiatrically ill older members of society. Nursing home placement is a drastic, restrictive, and costly intervention, and it is one of the most difficult decisions that adult protective services workers and elder abuse field workers face. One of the first articles published on outcomes of elder abuse and neglect was in the 1970s. The authors found that by being referred to adult protective services, elderly persons were more likely to be institutionalized [67]. One of the troubling findings of this study was that a system intended to protect the health and independence of the vulnerable elderly population was causing institutionalization. Others have suggested that services use rather than adult protective services use may be the reason for increased probability of nursing home placement. McFall and Miller [68], using the National Long Term care survey, found that use of community services was an independent predictor of nursing home admission. Whitlatch et al [69] found that receiving respite assistance among caregivers predicted nursing home placement. Due to the growing reporting of elder abuse and neglect cases, adult protective services worker's case loads have increased dramatically. In the absence of comprehensive community services and supports for the victims of elder abuse and neglect, adult protective service workers may feel pressured to solve difficult situations through nursing home placement [70].

Lachs et al [71] linked the well-established, community-based cohort of older adults (New Haven Established Population for Epidemiologic Studies in the Elderly [EPESE] cohort) with adult protective services records. The cohort had been previously linked with a long-term care data registry in the state of Connecticut, permitting the certainty of nursing home placement records for all cohort members. This study found that abused and neglected elderly persons referred to adult protective services is a predictor of nursing home placement, even after adjusting for other variables known to be associated with institutionalization in the older population. Variables accounted for were age, gender, race, education, income, and the number of chronic conditions (eg, arthritis, stroke, diabetes, and hip fracture). Other variables used in the analysis included any presence of ADL impairment, social ties, and resources for emotional support. Patients with verified mistreatment had a hazard ratio (HR) of 4.02 (95% confidence interval [CI], 2.50–6.47) and verified self-neglect when compared with those without verified mistreatment (HR, 5.23, 95% CI, 4.07–6.72). When compared with a prior study [72], ADL and cognitive impairment conferred a risk of placement of between 2-fold and 3-fold, which is far lower than the 4- to 5-fold risk conferred by elder mistreatment and self-neglect in this EPESE cohort.

From the adult protective services perspective, nursing home placement is not necessarily a terrible outcome. Nursing home placement can result in dramatic improvements in the quality of life. It takes frail elderly persons out of the abusive and neglectful environments and puts the patients under the care of health care professionals. Many of the medical and psychologic issues can be addressed during this period, and therapy can be prescribed. Further research is needed to direct us further on this issue. Beginning in the 1950s, adult protective services have become widely recognized [73]. Current literature does not contain any systematic attempt to evaluate program outcomes or to examine unintended consequences of adult protective services intervention. Controlled studies on different outcomes of the adult protective services need to be conducted. The positive benefits of the adult protective services intervention must be scientifically documented to justify the possible risk of negative outcomes.

Mortality

Abuse and neglect of elderly persons is associated with increased mortality [74]. There are no clear case finding guidelines, diagnostic tests, or legal or medical system interventions in the area of abuse and neglect [75,76]. MacMillan et al [77] noted that some mistreated elderly persons worsened after admission to the hospital and that the majority rapidly deteriorated, with few living in the community after 3 years. They reported a mortality rate of 50% over 4 years. Baker [78] in 1976 painted an even bleaker picture. He noted that 25% of elderly persons died within the first 3 weeks after admission and that soon after admission patients became bewildered, restless, and unable to report their needs except to express a desire to go home. He also noted an increasing prevalence of apathy, diminished appetite, an onset of incontinence, and an increase in the frequency of falls. Other studies have noted that in patients admitted to a hospital with a diagnosis of self-neglect, the mortality rates were high, especially for women, who experienced a 46% mortality rate [79]. Roe [80] reported 12% mortality within 3 weeks of admission and long-term inpatient expected mortality of 36%. The majority of those patients admitted to the hospital were discharged home and while in the hospital seemed to have a good quality of life. It seems justifiable in these cases to encourage admission to the hospital where there is a good chance of recovery and an added quality of life to what years or months remain. Wrigley and Cooney [81] found that within a 2-year period, 41% of patients admitted to an inpatient psychiatric unit returned home, 34% were in continuing care in a nursing home, and 18% died.

Lachs et al [14] investigated the independent contribution of reported elder abuse and neglect to all-cause mortality in an observed cohort of community-dwelling older adults. In the first 9 years after cohort inception, they found that elderly protective services had seen 72% for self-neglect, 17% for neglect, 5.7% for physical abuse, and 4.5% for financial exploitation. At the end of the 13-year follow-up period from the cohort inception, cohort members seen for elder mistreatment at any time during the follow-up had poorer survival (9%) than those seen for self-neglect (17%) or other noninvestigated cohort members (40%). In a pooled logistic regression that adjusted for demographic characteristics, chronic diseases, functional status, social networks, cognitive status, and depressive symptoms, the risk of death remained elevated.

A 10-year retrospective case review of morbidity and mortality among elders was conducted at a State Medical Examiner's Office serving a major metropolitan region in Kentucky and Indiana [82]. The study addressed medical-legal autopsies and examination of living subjects pursuant to a clinical forensic medicine program. The authors presented 74 postmortem cases in which 52 deaths were attributed to a homicidal act and 22 deaths were suspicious for neglect. Of the 22 living victims of elder abuse and neglect, 19 cases constituted physical or sexual assault, and three individuals suffered from neglect. Furthermore, 81.8% of the neglect cases had physical injuries, including abrasions and contusions, and 95.4% of the neglect cases revealed decubitus ulcers. The finding of decubitus ulcers should alert the health care professionals of potential neglect. Decubitus ulcers represent a significant source of morbidity and mortality in the frail elderly population [83]. A 6-fold increase in mortality has been linked to decubitus ulcers that have failed to heal [84].

Suicide is common among elderly persons, although its relationship to elder abuse and neglect is unknown. The highest rate of suicide occurs in men in their eighties. Suicide in the elderly population is more than double the average of all ages. Suicide remains one of the 10 leading causes of death in the United States and continues to be under-reported. People over 65 are extremely successful at suicide: their attempts rarely fail, particularly among men, although, the suicide rates for older women are rising around the world [57].

Implications for health care professionals

Role of health care professionals

Health care professionals play a critical role in the detection and management of elder abuse and neglect. Physicians are frequently in contact with elderly patients and are ideally situated to detect abuse and neglect and to play a significant role in the detection, management, and prevention of elder abuse and neglect. Elder abuse and neglect may be difficult to identify unless there are obvious signs of physical injury. Without a higher index of suspicion, elder abuse and neglect goes unnoticed. Even when abuse and neglect is detected, management is often complex, and evidence of successful management is sparse [85]. Because of poor public awareness and a lack of clear public health or practice guidelines and other factors, only 21% of the reported cases of abuse and neglect that occurred in 1996 were substantiated by adult protective services [86].

Physicians report only a small portion of all cases of elder abuse and neglect. In a recent survey of adult protective service workers for the elderly population, physicians were ranked tenth among health care professionals and paraprofessionals in assisting identification of elder abuse and neglect [87]. Dong et al [88] examined the elder abuse and neglect cases in Connecticut over the last 10 years. Of the more than 50,000 cases reported to the adult protective services in Connecticut, physician reporting accounted for less than 1.5%. This is unfortunate because the physician may be the only person outside the family who sees the older adult on a regular basis, and he or she is uniquely qualified to order confirmatory diagnostic procedures such as blood tests or x-rays, to recommend hospital admission, or to authorize services such as home health care.

There is general agreement that health care professionals have an important role in identifying and preventing abuse and neglect. However, little is known of the context in which health care professionals know and understand the problem. In 1997, a British survey was conducted to determine whether primary care physicians reported suspected cases of abuse and neglect and identified patients at risk [89]. They examined the readiness of physicians in detecting and managing abuse and neglect of elders: 49% of physicians reported diagnosing the abuse of an older patient in the last 12 months, 37% reported knowing patients in situations that might place an older patient at risk of abuse, 70% felt they needed further education on dealing with elder abuse and neglect, and 16% had attended a training course relating to topics of elder abuse and neglect. A subsequent survey of 561 physicians demonstrated that only 14% had attended a training course about elder abuse, that only 19% were aware of local guidelines on elder abuse, and that 72% of physicians would find training or education helpful [90].

Many health care professionals are ignorant of state mandatory reporting laws or choose to disregard them. In a 1987 study in Alabama, only 24% of the responding physicians practicing in internal medicine, family practice, or general practice were aware of the channels of reporting abuse cases; however, 38% physicians reported having seen cases of elder abuse and neglect in their practice [91]. A national survey of ER physicians showed that 52% of physicians described elder abuse and neglect as prevalent but less so than spousal or child abuse. Only 31% of physicians reported having a written protocol for the reporting of elder abuse and neglect, and they were generally not familiar with applicable state laws. Twenty-five percent of physicians were able to recall educational content related to elder abuse and neglect during their residencies. Most physicians (74%) were not certain or did not believe that clear-cut medical definitions of elder abuse or neglect exist, and 92% of physicians did not believe that their states have sufficient resources to meet the needs of the elderly victims [8].

When elder abuse or neglect occurs or is suspected, physicians should notify the proper authorities, even though sometimes this may be intimidating and there may be many barriers to reporting. Opportunities for detection and intervention vary with the discipline and the site at which the abuse or neglect is encountered. Family physicians, general internists, and psychiatrists may have well-established relationships with older adults and their families that allow them to recognize potential abuse and neglect and to intervene before a catastrophic event occurs. In contrast, ER physicians routinely witness the effect of elder abuse and neglect that requires immediate action to ensure the patient's safety and prevent further harm. In many states, physicians are legally required to report suspected cases of elder abuse and neglect. Physicians are rarely penalized for not reporting, but it should be part of one's moral and professional responsibility [92]. Physicians can make a major contribution to the advancement of knowledge, practice, and policy with regard to elder abuse and neglect, as they have done with child abuse.

Barriers to health care professional reporting

Elder abuse and neglect is no exception to the general unwillingness among primary care physicians to address family violence in all its forms. Many barriers to the reporting of elder abuse have been recognized and often are the results of incomplete and flawed medical education systems. Health care professionals can contribute to cases of abuse and neglect going undetected. Physicians under-report, and they notify the appropriate authorities in only 1 of 13 cases they identify [93]. Many physicians feel uncomfortable and are resistant to discuss potential abuse and neglect with their patients [94]. Few medical school curricula have formal training in the detection of elder abuse and neglect and interviewing techniques for potential victims and abusers [95]. This feeling of discomfort is likely to be due primarily to a lack of knowledge.

There is a lack of public and professional awareness and a misconception that there is a need to have ample proof of abuse and neglect before reporting. There is lack of professional protocol for helping physicians report elder abuse and neglect [22,27,96]. Most hospitals have no protocol for identifying or addressing elder abuse and neglect. Moreover, even if a physician recognizes a case, he or she may not know the proper management involved. As a result, many physicians have no tools to maintain a high index of suspicion with their older patients to recognize cases of abuse and neglect. One study found that physicians, by self-report, did not know the prevalence of elder abuse and neglect and hence did not think of this as a potential problem they might encounter [97].

In a busy practice setting, physicians do not always have the time to conduct an in-depth interview separately with the victim and then with other family members. In the era of medical reform, there is pressure for physicians to see more patients in shorter periods of time. Our patients are getting older and frailer, and there are many new guidelines and screening tools for many other aspects of medical health care. In a busy practice or in the ER, it is difficult to initiate such a sensitive discussion in conjunction with taking care of their complicated and more immediate medical issues. Often, there is need to get other patients into the limited examination rooms, and there is a lack of space to have such sensitive discussions. Our medical reimbursement system does not compensate physicians for spending extra time with patients for such discussions. In a typical practice, with the time spent on one patient of abuse and neglect, a physician could have seen many other patients. One survey showed that the time element was the most pervasive and driving fear for health care professionals. It magnified the other barriers mentioned by the physicians in reporting suspected cases. Higher priority will likely be given to the organic causes of disease that can be expediently dealt with in the time frame that has emerged for medical practice.

Sugg et al [98] surveyed primary care physicians in Seattle, Washington to examine the barriers for reporting suspected cases of elder abuse and neglect.

They found that 71% of physicians said they were too busy to investigate domestic violence. Many used the phrase "opening Pandora's box" to illustrate their reluctance to explore this issue. Thirty-nine percent of physicians felt that their patients had a low risk of domestic violence because they had backgrounds similar to their physician's. More than 50% of physicians thought they would offend the patient if they ask about domestic violence, 55% thought they were ill prepared to deal with the issue, and 61% reported no training in domestic violence. Many physicians felt that patients are responsible for dealing with their family situation. The close identification of physicians with patients of their own socioeconomic background can generate a denial that leads to hazardous consequences. Abused and neglected patients from higher socioeconomic groups are not acknowledged because they are asked. Furthermore, the misconception that domestic violence is largely a product of poverty is perpetuated through discriminating questioning of lower socioeconomic groups. The fear of offending the patients is implanted in our cultural construct of privacy. Not wanting to overstep the bounds of privacy, yet acknowledging that elder abuse and neglect has medical implications, leaves the physician reluctant to approach the issue of elder mistreatment.

Some physicians felt that they had no influence because their tools were limited to medications or surgeries, which are inadequate approaches to fix abuse and neglect. Other physicians felt that they did have tools in the form of emotional support or appropriate referrals but were frustrated by their inability to influence whether a patient accepted what was offered [97]. This is an area where the deficit in training is most apparent. When physicians encounter instances of abuse and neglect, they may feel fruitless in their ability to intercede. There are difficulties to access the abused person, including refusal by the abuser to allow health care professionals to intervene in diagnosis or treatment of the abused or neglected elders. Often patients may deny that mistreatment has happened and may resist intervention and may fear that abusers may attempt to isolate them from the health care system. Detecting elder abuse and neglect is challenging because an abusive situation may present itself in a nonsuspicious way, such as diagnosis of dehydration or failure to thrive. Physicians often feel disappointed and inadequate in discussing intervention or an inability to change the victim's situation [99].

Health care professionals need to be educated on appropriate intervention strategies and need to become more aware of the expected time courses of changes. Effective intervention, especially at time of crisis, often requires the introduction of law enforcement authorities into family affairs, an action that health care professionals usually are not at ease in taking. Physicians may show discomfort in confronting the alleged perpetrator and fear that the abuser will retaliate against the victim. Fear of litigation can make many physicians reluctant to ask questions about potential abuse and neglect. The physician often is in an uncomfortable position between protecting confidentiality, serving as an advocate for the elderly patient, and needing to collaborate with the family and often the abuser. The law usually is an ally in diagnosis and management of elder abuse and neglect, but physicians often are unfamiliar with legal aspects of elder mistreatment.

Effective strategies and interventions

Health care professional intervention in cases of elder abuse and neglect is a multidimensional undertaking. A first step in successful intervention is for the health care professional to examine his or her attitudes toward elderly abuse and neglect. When the health care professionals acknowledge that the phenomenon exists and have dealt with negative feelings toward aging or observe that elder abuse and neglect is possible in any family, then effective intervention can take place. The field of child abuse has taught us that the process of raising awareness and advocacy among health care professionals is essential to the advancement of knowledge and development of clinical guidelines and protocols.

There is the necessity for physicians to be aware that elder abuse and neglect exists and to be able to recognize the potential risk factors and symptoms. Education on elder abuse is best distributed across the medical student curriculum in preclinical and clinical courses and clerkships, especially those in the adult primary care disciplines [65]. There are opportunities to introduce the subjects of elder abuse and neglect in preclinical courses in the public health sciences, in social and community medicine, psychiatry, clinical medicine rotations, and geriatrics courses. Clinical electives in geriatrics should include classroom and experiential learning in elder abuse and neglect. Rotations in medicine, psychiatry, family medicine, and gynecology can include materials on elder abuse and neglect in case-based formats, lectures, or bedside teaching. The importance of educational initiatives in family violence including elder abuse and neglect should not be underestimated. The more we inquire into the phenomenon of family violence, the more we discover its extent, its severity, and its reality.

Jones et al [8] surveyed a group of physicians of whom most felt that elder abuse and neglect should be a part of in-service training for all ED staff, that standardized reporting procedures or guidelines are needed, that routine screening for elder abuse and neglect among elder patients should be instituted, and that a medical social worker should be available for the ED at all times. Other recommendations include ways to improve professional awareness of elder abuse and neglect through continuing medical education program, training videos, and seminars for law enforcement and emergency medical services staff. It is of major concern for educators that only 25% of emergency medicine residency graduates surveyed could recall any educational content pertaining to elder abuse and neglect during their residencies. Academic medical centers should take a leading role in promoting awareness and increase services at the local and state level. State and national medical societies need to make physicians aware of existing state laws, especially those regarding mandatory reporting, risk of liability, confidentiality, competency, and patient self-determination.

Clinics and hospitals should have guidelines to determine what information is necessary to assess and report cases of elder abuse and neglect. A health care professional is more likely to question an elderly patient's bruise if he or she has training in detecting mistreatment and feels comfortable with a protocol for identifying and reporting suspected abuse and neglect [100]. Although several excellent protocols are available [9,101,102], none has been tested extensively for its reliability and validity. Anetzberger et al [103] described a 2-year collaborative project in Cleveland, Ohio, that improved the reporting and management of potential and suspected elder abuse situations involving persons with dementia. An educational curriculum for cross training, screening tools, and referral protocols were developed and tested for health care professionals, staff, and volunteers in adult protective services with great success.

Responsible physicians should be familiar with the various forms of interventions that are available. These include the assistance of adult protective services or hospitalization and an alternative safe haven in cases of emergency. In non-emergency cases, collaborations with social workers and other professional agencies are crucial. Other strategies that have been postulated by physicians to be helpful include a single agency to call, a directory of services, a list of resource people, educational packages, guidelines for detection and management, reimbursement for time spent on legal matters, continuing education, revision of fee structures, and a central library of resources on elder abuse [27]. Increasing awareness at the local level of resources to help assess and manage elder abuse and neglect is a high priority. Lack of reimbursement for time spent on legal matters and the present fee structures were identified as barriers to effective management.

Elder abuse and neglect resource packages for use in clinical practice and guidelines or protocols for detecting and managing elder abuse were also identified as potentially valuable. Physicians who had attended continuing medical education courses on elder abuse and neglect were more likely to detect and report the mistreatment. The implication is that the continuing medical education courses may improve knowledge in this area [104]. Four models of effective educational collaborations with community-based service agencies demonstrate that learners from multiple levels of varied health care professional training programs are able to gain important experiences in geriatric care, particularly issues of elder abuse and neglect [105].

As a supporter to patient and caregiver, the physician should educate them regarding the aging process and the needs of the elderly patient and should offer guidance in cases of conflict between the elder and caregiver. Home visits offer the opportunity to provide valuable information about the care for and unmet needs of elderly patients. If physicians take a constructive role through educating and supporting caregivers of older patients, many of the causes of elder abuse and neglect could be eliminated. The health care setting has a vital role as a place of refuge for abused and neglected elderly people and gives health care workers an opportunity to identify abuse and neglect before it progresses [106]. The Journal of the American Medical Association Council recommends that physicians facing cases of elder abuse and neglect should be able to institute measures needed to prevent further injury, provide medical evaluation and treatment of injuries resulting from abuse and neglect, remain objective and nonjudgmental, attempt to establish or maintain a therapeutic alliance with the family, and report all suspected cases of elder abuse and neglect in accordance with local statutes [107]. Physicians should also encourage the development and use of supportive community resources that provide in-home services, respite care, and stress reduction within high-risk families.

No one person or profession should be solely responsible for the management of elder abuse and neglect. Therefore, a multidisciplinary team of caretakers from the medical, social services, mental health, and legal professions should be used whenever possible to achieve a clearly specified set of goals. These goals may include coordination, diagnosis or identification, prevention, treatment, consultation, and education. Elder abuse and neglect as a public health issue is in its early years and continues to evolve. Beyond providing clinical expertise, the physician can play an important role in encouraging and participating in research relating to elder abuse and neglect. The amount of rigorous scientific investigation about elder abuse and neglect has been minimal, especially when compared with the number of scientific investigations on child abuse performed during the same period [108]. Systematic prospective research is needed in most of areas related to elder abuse and neglect. Training and education need to be grounded in rigorous research-based knowledge about risk factors. There is a desperate need for outcomes research to effectively detect elder abuse and neglect and instill management protocols and most effective techniques.

Health care professionals first became aware of the cruelty of child abuse, which triggered a compassionate and outraged response. In the current society, voices of the older victims of abuse and neglect are being heard. There is an epidemic of elder abuse and neglect, especially with the growth of an increasingly frail and aging population that will need the care of a decreasing relative proportion of middle-aged children who will be split between the needs of their own children and those of their elderly family members. There is never a more urgent time for health care professionals to prepare to deal with such an epidemic problem.

Summary

Recognition of elder abuse and neglect among health care professionals has been a relatively recent phenomenon. Each year, millions of elderly persons suffer as the result of abuse and neglect. Their quality of life is severely jeopardized in the form of worsened functional status and progressive dependency, poorly rated self-health, and feelings of helplessness and from the vicious cycle of social isolation, stress, and further psychologic decline. Other medical implications of abuse and neglect include higher health system use in the form of frequent ER visits, higher hospitalization, and higher nursing home placement; most importantly, it is an independent predictor for higher mortality. Physicians are well situated for detecting and reporting suspected cases and for taking care of the frail elders who are victims of abuse and neglect, but there are many barriers on the individual level, and there is a broader need for system change. Through education, training, and reinforcement, there are strategies to get health care professionals more involved and provide effective management protocols and guidelines for us to advocate for our patients in the current epidemic of elder abuse and neglect.

References

[1] Tatara T. Summaries of national elder abuse data: an exploratory study of state statistics. Washington, Dca: National Aging Resource Center on Elder Abuse; 1990.

[2] Tatara T. Elder abuse. In: Edeards RL, editor. Encyclopedia of social work. 19th edition. Washington, DC: NASW Press; 1995. p. 834–42.

[3] US House of Representatives. Select Committee on Aging. Elder abuse: decades of shame and inaction. Washington, DC: Government Printing Office; 1990.

[4] Brownell P, Welty A, Brennan M. Elder abuse and neglect. Available at: www.aging.state.ny.us/explore/project2015/artabuse.htm. Accessed June 4, 2004.

[5] Pillemer KA, Finkelhor D. The prevalence of elder abuse: a random sample survey. Geronotologist 1988;28:51–7.

[6] Pang WS. Elder abuse: under-recognized and under-reported. Singapore Med J 2000;41: 567–70.

[7] Paris B. Abuse and neglect: so prevalent yet so elusive. Geriatrics 2003;58:10.

[8] Jones JS, Veenstra TR, Seamon JP, et al. Elder mistreatment: national survey of emergency physicians. Ann Emerg Med 1997;30:473–9.

[9] Aravanis SC, Adelman RD, Breckman R, et al. Diagnostic and treatment guidelines on elder abuse and neglect. Arch Fam Med 1993;2:371–88.

[10] Lachs MS, Pillemer K. Abuse and neglect of elderly persons. N Engl J Med 1995;332:437–43.

[11] Hamburger L, Saunders D, Hover M. Prevalence of domestic violence in community practice and rate of physician inquiry. Fam Med 1992;24:283–7.

[12] McCauley J, Kern DE, Kolodner K. The "battering syndrome": prevalence and clinical characteristics of domestic violence in primary care internal medicine practice. Ann Intern Med 1995;123:737–46.

[13] Watts C, Zimmerman C. Violence against women: global scope and magnitude. Lancet 2002; 359:1232–7.

[14] Lachs MS, Williams CS, O'Brien S, et al. The mortality of elder mistreatment. JAMA 1998; 280:428–32.

[15] Levine JM. Elder neglect and abuse: a primer for primary care physicians. Geriatrics 2003;58:37–44.

[16] Dyer CB, Pavlik VN, Murphy KP, et al. The high prevalence of depression and dementia in elder abuse and neglect. J Am Geriatr Soc 2000;48:205–8.

[17] American Medical Association White Paper on Elderly Health. Report of the Council on Scientific Affairs. Arch Intern Med 1990;150:2459–72.

[18] Mouton CP, Rodabough RJ, Rovi SLD, et al. Prevalence and 3 year incidence of abuse among postmenopausal women. Am J Public Health 2004;94:605–12.

[19] Burston GR. Granny-battering. BMJ 1975;3:592.

[20] Dobrin A, Wiersema B, Loftin C. Statistical handbook on violence in America. Phoenix (AZ): Oryx Press; 1996.

[21] Rosenblatt DE, Kyung-Hwan C. Reporting mistreatment of older adults: the role of physicians. J Am Geriatr Soc 1996;44:65–70.

[22] Clark-Daniel CL. Abuse and neglect of the elderly: are emergency department personnel aware of mandatory reporting laws? Ann Emerg Med 1990;19:970–7.

[23] Jogerst GJ, Daly JM, Brinig MF, et al. Domestic elder abuse and law. Am J Public Health 2003;93:2131–6.

[24] Hogstel MO, Curry LC. Elder abuse revisited. J Gerontol Nursing 1999;25:10–8.

[25] Kane RA, Kane RL. Assessing the elderly: a practical guide to measurement. Lexington (MA): LexingtonBooks; 1981.

[26] Homer AC, Gilleard C. Abuse of the elderly people by their carers. BMJ 1990;301:1359–62.

[27] Kleinschmidt KC. Elder abuse: a review. Ann Emerg Med 1997;30:463–72.

[28] Coyne AC, Reichman WE, Berbig LJ. The relationship between dementia and elder abuse. Am J Psychiatry 1993;150:643–6.

[29] Podnieks E. National survey on abuse of the elderly in Canada. J Elder Abuse Neglect 1992;4:5–58.

[30] Villomare E, Bergman J. Elder abuse and neglect: a guide for practitioner and policy makers. San Francisco (CA); National Paralegal Institute; 1981.

[31] Jones JS, Holstege C, Holstege H. Elder abuse and neglect: understanding the causes and potential risk factors. Am J Emerg Med 1997;15:579–83.

[32] Steinmetz SK, Amsden DJ. Dependent elders, family stress, and abuse. In: Brubaker TH, editor. Family relationships in later life. Beverly Hills (CA): Sage Publications; 1983. p. 173–92.

[33] Cantor M. Family and community: changing roles in an aging society. Gerontologist 1991; 31:337–46.

[34] Idler EL. Self-assessed health and mortality: a review of studies. Int Rev Health Psychol 1992;1:33–54.

[35] Liang J. Self-reported health among aged adults. Gerontologist 1986;41:248–60.

[36] WHO/INPEA. Missing voices: views of older persons on elder abuse. Available at: www.who.int/hpr/ageing/MissingVoices.pdf. Accessed June 4, 2004.

[37] Seligman MEP. Helplessness. San Francisco: Freeman Publishing; 1975.

[38] Bookin D, Dunkle RE. Elder abuse: issues for the practitioner. Social Casework 1985; Jan:3–12.

[39] Longres JF. Self neglect and social control: a modest test of an issue. J Gerontol Soc Work 1994;22:3–20.

[40] Lau EE, Kosberg JI. Abuse of the elderly by informal care provider. Aging 1979:10–5.

[41] Moon A, Williams O. Perceptions of elder abuse and help seeking patterns among African-American, Caucasian American, and Korean-American elderly women. Gerontologist 1993; 33:386–95.

[42] Faulkner LR. Mandating the reporting of suspected cases of elder abuse: an inappropriate, ineffective and ageist response to the abuse of older adults. Fam Law Q 1982;16:69–91.

[43] Breckman R, Adelman R. Strategies for helping victims of elder mistreatment. Beverly Hills (CA): Sage Publications; 1998.

[44] Dohrenwend BS, Dohrenwend BP. Stressful life events: their nature and effects. New York: Wiley; 1974.

[45] Linsky AA, Straus MA. Social stress in the United States: links to regional patterns in crime and illness. Dover (MA): Auburn House; 1986.

[46] Mathews KA, Glass DC. Type-A behavior, stressful life events and coronary heart disease. In: Hohrenwend BS, Hohrenwend BP, editors. Stressful life events and their context. New York: Wiley; 1981.

[47] Harrell R, Toronjo CH, McLaughlin J, et al. How geriatricians identify elder abuse and neglect. Am J Med Sci 2002;323:34–8.

[48] Linsky AA, Bachman R, Straus MA. Stress, culture, and aggression. New Haven (CT): Yale University; 1995.

[49] Nahmiash D. Powerlessness and abuse and neglect of older adults. J Elder Abuse Neglect 2004;14:21–47.

[50] Ward D. Ageism and the abuse of older people in health and social care. Br J Nurs 2000;9:560–3.

[51] Okun MA, Melichar JF, Hill MD. Negative daily events, positive and negative social ties, and psychological distress among older adults. Gerontologist 1990;30:193–9.

[52] Vinocur AD, van Ryn M. Social support and undermining in close relationships: their independent effects on the mental health of unemployed persons. J Personal Soc Psychol 1993; 65:350–9.

[53] Rock K. The negative side of social interaction: impact on psychological well-being. J Personal Soc Psychol 1984;46:1097–108.

[54] Childs HW, Hayslip B, Radika LM, et al. Young and middle-aged adult's perception of elder abuse. Gerontologist 2000;40:75–85.

[55] Neville P, Boyle A, Baillon S. A descriptive survey of acute bed usage for dementia care in old age psychiatry. Int J Geriatr Psychiatry 1999;14:348–54.

[56] Miller M. Suicide after 60: the final alternative. New York: Springer; 1979.

[57] McIntosh JL, Hubbard RW. Indirect self destructive behavior among the elderly: a review with case examples. J Gerontol Soc Work 1988;13:37–48.

[58] Mouton CP, Espino DV. Problem-orientated diagnosis: health screening in older women. Am Fam Physician 1999;59:1835–42.

[59] Spaite DW, Criss EA, Valenzuela TD, et al. Geriatric injury: an analysis of prehospital demographics, mechanisms, and patterns. Ann Emerg Med 1990;19:1418–21.

[60] Carmel S, Anson O, Levin M. Emergency department utilization: a comparative analysis of older adults, old and old-old patients. Aging Clin Exp Res 1990;2:387–93.

[61] Lowenstein SR, Crescenzi CA, Kern DC, et al. Care of the elderly in the emergency department. Ann Emerg Med 1986;15:528–35.

[62] McKinney EA, Young AT. Changing patient populations: considerations for service delivery. Health Soc Work 1985;10:292–9.

[63] Select Committee on Aging, House of Representatives, Subcommittee on Human Services. Elder abuse: an assessment of the federal response. Washington, DC: 1989.

[64] Lachs MS, Williams CS, O'Brien S, et al. ED use by older victims of family violence. Ann Emerg Med 1997;30:448–54.

[65] Jones JS. Elder abuse and neglect: responding to a national problem. Ann Emerg Med 1994;23:845–8.

[66] Fulmer T, Firpo A, Guadagno L, et al. Themes from a grounded theory analysis of elder neglect assessment by experts. Gerontologist 2003;43:745–52.

[67] Blenkner M. A research and demonstration of protective services. Soc Casework 1971;52: 483–97.

[68] McFall S, Miller BH. Caregiver burden and nursing home admission of frail elderly person. J Gerontol Soc Sci 1992;47:S73–9.

[69] Whitlatch CJ, Feinberg L, Stevens EJ. Predictors of institutionalization for persons with Alzheimer's disease and the impact on family caregivers. J Mental Health Aging 1999;5: 275–88.

[70] Wolf RS, Pillemer K. Helping elderly victims: the realty of elder abuse. New York: Columbia Univeristy Press; 1989.

[71] Lachs MS, Williams CS, O'Brien S, et al. Adult protective service use and nursing home placement. Gerontologist 2002;42:734–9.

[72] Foley DJ, Ostfeld AM, Branch LG, et al. The risk of nursing home admission in three communities. J Aging Health 1992;4:155–73.

[73] Mixson PM. Adult protective services perspective. Journal of Elder Abuse and Neglect 1995;7:69–87.

[74] Ortmann C, Fechner G, Bajanowski T, Brinkmann B. Fatal neglect of the elderly. Int J Legal Med 2001;114:191–3.

[75] Fulmer TT, O'Malley TA. The difficulty of defining abuse and neglect. In: Fulmer TT, O'Malley TA, editors. Inadequate care the elderly. New York: Springer; 1987. p. 13–24.

[76] Loue SL. Elder abuse and neglect in medicine and law: the need to reform. J Leg Med 2001;22:159–209.

[77] MacMillan D, Shaw P. Senile breakdown in standards of personal and environmental cleanliness. BMJ 1966;2:227–9.

[78] Baker A. Slow euthanasia-or 'she will be better off in hospital'. BMJ 1976;2:571–2.

[79] Clark A, Mankikar G, Gray I. Diogenese syndrome: a clinical study of gross self-neglect in old age. Lancet 1975;i:366–8.

[80] Roe P. Self neglect. Age Aging 1977;6:192–4.

[81] Wrigley M, Cooney C. Diogenes syndrome: an Irish Series. Irish J Psychol Med 1992;9:37–41.

[82] Shields LBE, Hunsaker DM, Hunsaker JC. Abuse and neglect: a ten year review of mortality and morbidity in our elders in a large metropolitan area. J Forensic Sci 2004;49:1–6.

[83] Emanuele JA, Katz T, Levien DH. Pressures sores: how to prevent and treat them. Postgrad Med 1992;91:113–20.

[84] Allman RM, Laprade CA, Noel LB, et al. Pressures sores among hospitalized patients. Ann Intern Med 1986;105:337–42.

[85] Canadian Task Force on the Periodic Health Examination. periodic health examination, 1994 update: 4 Secondary prevention of elder abuse and mistreatment. CMAJ 1994;151: 1413–20.

[86] National Center on Elder Abuse. The national elder abuse incidence study. Washington, DC: American Public Human Services Association; 1998.

[87] Blakey BE, Dolon R. The relative contributions of occupation groups in the discovery and treatment of elder abuse and neglect. J Gerontol Soc Work 1991;17:183–99.

[88] Dong X, Lachs MS, Tinette ME. Reporting patterns of elder abuse and neglect in Connecticut: an analysis of statewide database from 1992 to 2001. J Am Geriatr Soc 2002;50:147.

[89] McCreadie C, Bennett G, Tinker A. General practitioners knowledge and experience of the abuse of older people in the community: report of an exploratory research study in the inner-London borough of Tower Hamlets. Br J Gen Pract 1998;48:1687–8.

[90] McCreadie C, Bennett G, Gilthorpe MS, et al. Elder abuse: do general practitioners know or care? J R Soc Med 2000;93:67–71.

[91] Daniels RS, Baumhover LA, Clark-Daniels CL. Physician's mandatory reporting of elder abuse. Gerontologist 1989;29:321–7.

[92] Ahmed M, Lachs MS. Elder abuse and neglect: what physicians can and should do. Clev Clin J Med 2002;69:801–8.

[93] Colin M. Silent suffering: a case study of elder abuse and neglect. J Am Geriatr Soc 1998; 46:885–8.

[94] Cammer Paris BE. Violence against elderly people. Mount Sinai J Med 1996;63:97–100.

[95] Hazzard W. Elder abuse: definitions and implications for medical education. Acad Med 1995; 70:979–81.

[96] Swagerty Jr DL, Takahashi PY, Evans JM. Elder mistreatment. Am Fam Physician 1999; 59:2804–8.

[97] Clark-Daniels CL, Daniels RS, Baumhover LA. Physician's and nurse's response to abuse of the elderly: a comparative study of two surveys in Alabama. J Elder Abuse Neglect 1989;1: 57–72.

[98] Sugg NK, Inui T. Primary care physician's response to domestic violence: opening Pandora's box. JAMA 1992;267:3157–61.

[99] Marshall CE, Benton D, Brazier JM. Elder abuse: using clinical tools to identify clues of mistreatment. Geriatrics 2000;55:42–53.

[100] McNamara RM, Rousseau E, Sanders A. Geriatric emergency medicine: a survey of practicing emergency physicians. Ann Emerg Med 1992;21:796–801.

[101] Jones J, Dougherty J, Schelble D. Emergency department protocol for the diagnosis and evaluation of geriatric abuse. Ann Emerg Med 1988;17:1006–15.

[102] Mount Sinai/Victim Services Agency Elder Abuse Project. Elder mistreatment guidelines for health care professionals: detection, assessment, and intervention. New York: 1988.

[103] Anetzberger GJ, Palmisano BR, Sanders M, et al. A model intervention for elder abuse and dementia. Gerontologist 2000;40:492–7.

[104] Krueger P, Patterson C. Detection and managing elder abuse: challenges in primary care. CMAJ 1997;157:1095–100.

[105] Heath JM, Dyer CB, Kerzner LJ, et al. Four models of medical education about elder mistreatment. Acad Med 2002;77:1101–6.

[106] Malouf P, Paulus F. Maintaining older people's dignity and autonomy in healthcare settings: elder abuse is both community and healthcare issue. BMJ 2001;323:340.

[107] Council on Scientific Affairs. Council report: elder abuse and neglect. JAMA 1987;257: 966–71.

[108] Wolf RS. Elder abuse: ten years later. J Am Geriatr Soc 1988;36:758–62.

ELSEVIER
SAUNDERS

CLINICS IN
GERIATRIC
MEDICINE

Clin Geriatr Med 21 (2005) 315–332

Dementia and Elder Abuse

Maria R. Hansberry, MD[a,c,*], Elaine Chen, BS[b],
Martin J. Gorbien, MD, FACP[a,c]

[a]Department of Internal Medicine, Section of Geriatric Medicine, Rush University Medical Center,
710 South Paulina Street, Chicago, IL 60612, USA
[b]Rush Medical College, 600 South Paulina Street, Chicago, IL 60612, USA
[c]Section of Geriatric Medicine, Rush University Medical Center, 710 South Paulina Street,
Chicago, IL 60612, USA

Dementia is a clinical syndrome characterized by acquired persistent losses of cognitive function in multiple areas. The etiologies for dementia are broad and include degenerative, vascular, infectious, neoplastic, traumatic, toxic, metabolic, or psychiatric disorders [1]. Alzheimer disease (AD) is the most prevalent form of dementia, accounting for approximately 50% of progressive dementias [2]. In 2000, approximately 4.5 million Americans were affected by AD, and AD is projected to affect 13 million Americans by 2050 [3].

As the geriatric population grows, with the over-85 group growing the most rapidly, the number of Americans with dementia will increase. Estimates of the prevalence of AD range from 5% to 10% of all Americans older than 65. Studies consistently show that incidence and prevalence of dementia increases exponentially with age, doubling every 5 years up to age 90 or 95 [4–6]. The prevalence of dementia in the nursing home is higher than in the general population: More than 50% of nursing home residents have dementia [7].

Progression of dementia leads to loss of function in memory, performance of familiar tasks, language, orientation, judgment, abstract thinking, mood, and behavior. Due to the multifactorial etiologies of dementia, there is no one clas-

---

* Corresponding author. Department of Internal Medicine, Section of Geriatric Medicine, Rush University Medical Center, 710 South Paulina Street, Chicago, IL 60612.

E-mail address: maria_r_hansberry@rush.edu (M.R. Hansberry).

sical, clinical course. However, each cause of dementia is typified by characteristic presentations and progressions. For example, vascular dementia results from cerebrovascular ischemia and often presents with a fluctuating and incremental course. Pick disease, a frontotemporal dementia, is associated with language problems, loss of personal and social awareness, and disordered executive function, although memory and cognition are relatively preserved [8,9].

AD is typified by three stages: mild, moderate, and severe. Symptoms in the mild stage begin with minor changes in memory and language. Onset of behavioral changes, such as increasing agitation, marks moderate stage dementia. AD is commonly complicated by psychosis and depression, which is often associated with psychomotor retardation and decreased decisional capacity. In severe disease, all intellectual abilities are markedly impaired, and motor dysfunction emerges. Patients in the terminal phases of any dementia generally become incontinent and lose the ability to walk. Special care must be taken to protect skin integrity, prevent urinary tract infections and aspiration, and maintain hydration and nutrition [1]. A commonly cited prognosis for AD is between 3 and 20 years from time of diagnosis. Some patients with AD have been reported to decline from full cognition to death in less than 1 year, whereas others may plateau and survive for many years after diagnosis [10]. The inevitable decline in cognitive and physical function over months to years and subsequent dependence on others to meet daily needs yields an increasingly vulnerable population of elders with dementia.

Many therapies are available to treat the symptoms of dementia and its complications. Perhaps the most essential component of the care of a dementia patient is education of the patient and family. Ideally, the care of elders with dementia is coordinated by a multidisciplinary team. Input from nurses, social workers, physical and occupational therapists, clinical psychologists, and the primary physician are integrated to deliver optimal care of the patient. It is important to educate the early-stage dementia patient and the caregiver about anticipated assistance with personal needs and management of disruptive behaviors. It is perhaps more important to educate the patient, caregiver, and family about the expected clinical course for the disease and to ensure understanding of the complications that arise as dementia progresses.

In addition to education, behavioral and environmental manipulations and medications are instrumental to the care of the dementia patient. Behavioral and environmental therapies that have been shown to be beneficial include providing a fixed environment, regular schedules, and clocks to help orient the patient. Exercise training has been shown to improve physical health and decrease depression in AD patients. The residence should be organized so that wandering is permissible and safe. Nonpharmacologic measures such as these are first-line treatments for confusion and agitation in dementia patients. Advantages of these methods are lower financial cost and minimization of hazardous drug side effects and interactions of drug therapy. A primary disadvantage to these methods is the potential increased physical and emotional burden they pose to the caregiver [8,10,11].

As an adjunct to nonpharmacologic therapies, a variety of medications are available to treat comorbid behavior disturbances and mood disorders associated with dementia. Atypical antipsychotics, such as risperidone and olanzapine, are the preferred treatment for agitation with or without psychosis, hallucinations, and paranoid delusions. Anti-epileptic drugs have been used for paroxysmal and aggressive behavior without psychosis. Sedatives, such as benzodiazepines, are discouraged due to the risks of oversedation, paradoxic agitation, falls, and decreased memory. In the setting of other depressive features, agitation may respond well to low-dose trazodone and selective serotonin reuptake inhibitors [2,8].

Cholinesterase inhibitors, such as donepezil, rivastigmine, galantamine, and tacrine, have been used to treat mild to moderate disease and are the standard of care. Decrease in cognitive decline and decreased neuropsychiatric symptoms and improved behavior and function have been demonstrated in patients. Recently, memantine, an NMDA inhibitor, has been approved for patients with moderate to severe AD, showing reduced functional, behavioral, and cognitive decline. Trials are promising for the use of memantine in mild to moderate disease to preserve cognitive function [2,8,12].

Physical restraints are sometimes used to manage behavior that is deemed threatening to the safety of the patient or others. Mechanical restraints are devices, often cloth or leather, applied to individuals to inhibit free movement. Dementia patients are especially prone to unsteadiness, disruptiveness, agitation, and wandering; these behaviors are considered harmful by health care personnel and result in restraint use. The use of physical restraints has been controversial, and data are inadequate regarding the frequency and effectiveness of use. Following OBRA '87, interventions have been underway to decrease restraint use in nursing homes [13–15].

Elder abuse

Elder abuse is a problem affecting an estimated 1% to 12% of American elders living in the community, with 32 per 1000 being the most frequently cited estimate [16–18]. Data regarding elder abuse are difficult to find and interpret because elder abuse is a relatively recently recognized entity, has a wide variety of definitions from state to state, and is subject to cultural interpretation. Elder abuse may be domestic, taking place in the home of the abused or in the home of a caregiver, or it may be institutional, taking place in a residential facility for the elderly (eg, a nursing home). Elder abuse may be intentional (active) or unintentional (passive) [19]. Physical abuse is only one among many subtypes or elder abuse, which include psychologic abuse, financial abuse, sexual abuse, and neglect. Although these subtypes are discrete entities, they are often closely related and interdependent. In an extensive study, neglect was found to be the most common form of abuse, followed by psychologic abuse, financial exploitation, physical abuse, abandonment, and sexual abuse. In the home, two thirds of abusers are spouses and adult children [18].

Several theories have been proposed to explain the onset of elder abuse. So-cial learning of abusive behaviors, caregiver stress, social isolation of the victim, dependency between the victim and the abuser, and psychopathology of the abuser are commonly accepted theories [19–21]. The caregiver stress theory of abuse is the most frequently cited argument supporting a relationship between dementia and elder abuse. According to this theory, elder abuse is consequent to stresses that the caregiver experiences within the caregiving role or outside of it [20,22]. A poor premorbid relationship between caregiver and care recipient is a predictor of stress leading to abuse [23].

Many characteristics of the perpetrator and the victim have been cited as potential risk factors for elder abuse. A shared living arrangement lends itself to an increased risk of abuse due to the proximity of the abused and the abuser, and greater risk has been noted if the patient resides with immediate family but without a spouse [24]. Characteristics of the perpetrator that increase the risk of abuse include a history of mental illness, substance abuse, or dependence on the victim for financial assistance, housing, or other needs [25]. Perception of stress by the caregiver, not the stress level, was correlated with increased abuse [19]. Characteristics of the elder, including frailty, poor health, and functional impair-ments, have been shown to be associated with an increased probability of mistreatment, although these data are controversial [19,26]. An elder's aggressive behavior toward caregivers has been shown to increase the probability of physical abuse [24]. Elderly persons most susceptible to neglect were those in poorer health, more socially isolated and without contacts to call for help [25]. Because of the difficulties involved with studying elder abuse, many situations and factors may present as red flags for abuse but cannot be substantiated by the literature.

Dementia has been studied as a risk factor for elder abuse. Conflicting data exist regarding this relationship. An observational cohort study of 68 elderly patients in New Haven, Connecticut demonstrated that older age, minority status, poor social networks, and functional (but not cognitive) disability based on Mental Status Questionnaire errors were risk factors for abuse [27]. Conversely, a case control study of 142 elderly patients in Houston, Texas demonstrated a significantly higher prevalence of dementia among elder abuse victims [28]. One 9-year longitudinal study found an association between the new onset of cognitive impairment and elder abuse and neglect [26]. Several experts who have studied the profile of the elder abuse victim include cognitive impairment as a risk factor for abuse [17,20,21,29]. It can be speculated that with the increasing use of cholinesterase inhibitors and other pharmacologic treatments, dementia patients are living longer, thus prolonging their period of vulnerabil-ity to abuse.

Care of dementia patients at home

For most of the disease course, dementia patients are primarily cared for by first-degree relatives at home, usually a spouse (approximately 7%) or an adult child (approximately 50%); the remaining 43% of caregivers are other relatives or friends [30]. Dementia patients have a wide variety of care needs, far greater than their cohort without cognitive impairment. In a study comparing care for dementia and nondementia patients, it was shown that caregivers of dementia patients assist in significantly more activities than do caregivers of nondementia patients. Dementia patients required more assistance for each type of activity of daily living (eg, dressing, ambulating, bathing, using the toilet, feeding, and taking medication) than did nondementia patients. With respect to instrumental activities of daily living (eg, managing finances, groceries, housework, and transportation), dementia caregivers provided more care overall [30].

As their cognitive and functional decline progresses, dementia patients require more assistance. Needs that cannot be expressed due to memory and language difficulties, to decline in thought process and motor abilities need to be anticipated by the caregiver. Hydration and nutrition must be carefully monitored because patients may not recognize their own needs and may be unable to properly feed themselves. Patients often experience dysphagia and need extra assistance to ensure adequate intake and prevent aspiration. As patients lose mobility, turning and repositioning become necessary to minimize the risk of pressure ulcers. With assistance from health care providers, caregivers are responsible for managing the dementia patient's disruptive behavior, wandering, depression, psychosis, and aggression.

These burdens of care are among the constellation of factors that contribute to caregiver stress. Dementia is a progressive loss of cognitive function potentially, associated with aggressive behavior [23]. The stress of this circumstance is compounded if caregiver education regarding the progressive nature of dementia is lacking. Another source of caregiver stress is the situation of "generation inversion" that results when an individual cares for an elderly parent while attending to his own children, causing emotional and financial stress [31]. Caregiver stress has been associated with abuse by care recipient and the caregiver [32].

Caregiver depression has been cited as a significant factor in the incidence of severe family violence involving patients with AD, with violence defined to include acts of physical abuse committed by the caregiver or by the recipient of care [24]. Depression is reported at a higher rate among caregivers unable to cope with problematic behaviors [33]. Physical, emotional, and financial burdens have been reported at higher rates among caregivers of patients with dementia compared with those of patients without dementia [30]. Caregiving cost per patient has been estimated at $105 per month [30]. Caregivers who abuse provide care for more years, more hours per day, and for patients at lower functional levels. They have higher levels of burden and higher depression scores than a control group of nonabusers (Table 1) [22].

Elder abuse in the home takes many forms. The most frequent form of abuse in this population is self-neglect, defined as the failure to provide oneself the means to physical and psychiatric health. This finding is consistent with the pattern of abuse observed in the elderly population taken as a whole (Tables 2

Table 1
Patient abuse of caregiver

Variable	Yes		No		
	Mean	SD	Mean	SD	P value
Years of care	4.4	3.6	3.2	3.5	<.001
Hours of care/day	11.6	9.9	9.3	9.3	
Patient's functional status	3.4	0.8	3.0	0.8	<.001
Zarit Burden score	45.9	14.7	41.8	16.4	

Abbreviation: SD, standard deviation.

and 3) [20]. Three quarters of substantiated self-neglecting elders were found to have some degree of confusion [18]. Self-neglect is a multifaceted behavioral entity that involves the inability or refusal to adequately attend to one's health, safety, hygiene, nutrition, or social needs [34]. Self-neglect may stem from cognitive deficits attributable to dementia as a primary diagnosis or may be a symptom of depression, a comorbidity found to be significantly more prevalent in elderly abused patients than in age-matched control subjects [28]. Depression and cognitive impairment have been found to be independent predictors of self-neglect, and individuals with both types of symptoms had an enhanced risk of self-neglect. Self-neglect in the setting of dementia often reflects an inability to care for one's self, whereas self-neglect in the setting of depression often reflects a lack of willingness to care for oneself.

Decreased ability to communicate effectively can lead to anger, resentment, and frustration, resulting in highly conflicted relationships between the caregiver and the patient [33]. Aggressive behavior, which includes verbal outbursts, physical threats, and violence [24], is estimated to occur in approximately 57% to 67% of dementia patients and occurs most frequently during intimate care [33]. Severe violence by the patient toward the caregiver, including kicking, hitting, punching, biting, and threatening with or using a weapon, was reported in 15.8% of patients in 1 year [24]. One study showed that 26% of caregivers who were physically abused by patients directed abuse back toward their patients, as compared with 5% of those who were not abused by their patients [22]. It has been estimated that a person with AD is 2.25 times at greater risk for a physically abusive episode than a randomly sampled older person living in the community [24].

Cognitive impairment is recognized as a risk factor to financial exploitation, which is characterized by a misappropriation of assets by dishonest means [35]. The prevalence of elder abuse affects up to 12% of elders when financial abuse is included in the definition [35,36]. Financial exploitation may take the form of door-to-door scams, professional swindles, or, most commonly, theft by caregivers and family members. When managing money becomes a difficult task, elders who are cognitively impaired often turn to a trusted family member or friend for assistance with their finances. Elders with dementia become exceptionally vulnerable to coercion tactics leading to improper transfer of funds unknowingly signing checks and wills. Perpetrators may threaten dependent

Table 2
National estimates of the incidence of abuse, neglect, and self-neglect of persons 60 years and older, 1996 (unduplicated)

| | Estimated number of elderly persons[a] | | | (4) Total: columns (1) and (3) |
	(1) Reported by sentinels	(2) Reported to APS	(3) Reported to APS: substantiated only	
Total abuse, neglect, and Self-neglect (SE)	435,901 (114,887)	236,479 (34,298)	115,110 (20,326) 48.7%	551,011 (118,008)
Total abuse and neglect (SE)	378,982 (117,758)	151,408 (18,999)	70,942 (11,881) 46.9%	449,924 (119,512)
Abuse (SE)	355,218 (116,875)	95,761 (15,579)	47,069 (9,814) 49.2%	402,287 (116,084)
Neglect[b] (SE)	147,035 (52,290)	85,143 (12,966)	35,333 (6,706) 41.5%	182,368 (58,743)
Self-neglect (SE)	81,635 (21,966)	113,573 (28,907)	57,345 (15,350) 50.5%	138,980 (24,232)

Abbreviations: APS, Adult Protective Services; SE, standard error.
[a] Subtotals do not add to totals because more than one type of abuse was reported for some cases.
[b] Includes abandonment.
Data from The National Elder Abuse Incidence Study: final report. Washington, DC: Administration on Aging; 1998.

Table 3
Types of elder maltreatment substantiated by Adult Protective Services agencies

Maltreatment	Number of reports	Percentage[a]
Neglect	34,525	48.7
Emotional/psychologic abuse	25,142	35.4
Financial/material exploitation	21,427	30.2
Physical abuse	18,144	25.6
Abandonment	2560[b]	3.6
Sexual abuse	219[b]	0.3
Other	994[b]	1.4
Total incidents	70,942[c]	

[a] Estimated number of substantiated reports of domestic elder abuse with each type of maltreatment, 1996. Cases of self-neglect only are excluded.

[b] The confidence band for this number is wide relative to the size of the estimate. The true number may be close to zero or much larger than the estimate.

[c] Total incidents do not equal totals across abuse categories because more than one substantiated type of abuse was often reported for an incident.

elders with denial of basic necessities if the desired material is not granted. When cognition is sufficiently intact for the victim to recognize abuse, feelings of guilt, fear, embarrassment, and shame may contribute to the unwillingness of a victim to report episodes of financial exploitation. Psychologic abuse, including deception, intimidation, and threats, accompanies financial exploitation [35,37].

Care of dementia patients in nursing homes

When a dementia patient's care needs exceed the capabilities of caregivers at home, the elder may be placed in a nursing home. About 5% of persons age 65 and over reside in nursing homes at any given time, ranging from about 1% for those aged 65 to 74 to 20% for those over age 85. Approximately 45% of women and 28% of men will spend some part of their lives in a nursing home [38]. Because of the rapid growth of the over-85 segment of the population, the lifetime risk of nursing home use is expected to increase [39]. There are many predictors of nursing home placement, including advanced age, living alone, functional impairment, poverty, and lack of social support [40]. Incontinence, irritability, inability to walk, wandering, hyperactivity, and nocturnal behavioral problems are leading reasons for placement of dementia patients cited by caregivers [41]. Nursing home residents are in general more disabled than their cohorts who are living in the community, particularly with respect to their activities of daily living, and approximately half have some degree of dementia. Many dementia patients in long-term care settings suffer from several chronic medical conditions leading to even more limitations in physical and cognitive function and leaving them more dependent than dementia patients in the community [39,42,43].

Nursing home residents have been described as the most vulnerable members of society because they are dependent on the nursing facility for virtually all of their needs including food, medication, medical and dental care, and assistance with daily tasks [39]. Further, dementia patients in the nursing home continue the cognitive and functional decline that began before admission.

Risk factors for elder abuse in long-term care settings have been less extensively studied than for community-dwelling elders. Residents with behavioral symptoms, such as physical aggressiveness, are at higher risk for abuse by nursing home staff [44]. Some abusive behaviors by staff members are described as being reflexive or protective actions in response to patient aggression. Inadequate training, heavy workload, stressful working situations, staffing shortages, and overtime work are described as factors contributing to likelihood of abuse [39].

State nursing home ombudsman programs have received complaints of nursing home staff maltreatment for many years [45]. The true incidence and prevalence is unknown because abuse and neglect are suspected to be grossly under-reported. Facility staff and family members might be uncomfortable reporting abusive behavior regardless of assurances of confidentiality. Patients and family members might fear retaliation by nursing home staff or other caregivers. Potentially abused dementia patients are often poor candidates for interviews because information collected from them cannot be considered reliable [39,46].

Like those being cared for at home, dementia patients residing in nursing homes are at risk for several types of elder abuse. In one study of nursing homes, a random sample of nurses and nursing aides at 31 nursing homes in New Hampshire was interviewed. Of those interviewed, 36% and 81% of staff witnessed incidents of physical and psychologic abuse, respectively, and 10% admitted to committing acts of physical abuse. Physical abuse included excessively restraining patients, pushing, grabbing, slapping, kicking, and throwing things at patients. Forty percent of staff members admitted to more than one psychologically abusive act over the past year. Psychologically abusive actions most frequently constituted yelling at patients in anger but also included swearing at, isolating, and threatening patients [47].

Neglect of patients in nursing homes is more difficult to quantify. Neglect has been defined as the failure to provide goods and services necessary to avoid physical harm, mental anguish, or mental illness. It can also be thought of as failure of the responsible caretaker to provide services to maintain the elder's physical and mental health [26]. In surveys, up to 95% of nursing home residents who were interviewed reported that they had recently themselves experienced neglect or witnessed other residents being neglected [39]. Complaints included leaving residents wet or soiled with feces, shutting off call lights without providing assistance, not turning and repositioning residents, and not assisting residents with eating and drinking. Nursing and aide staff are also aware of the widespread nature of patient neglect, citing times of short staffing and shift changes as times when neglect is more likely to occur [39]. Self-neglect is harder to assess in the nursing home population than in the community-dwelling population because, whereas some elders can contribute to their own self-care, this capacity decreases over time among those with dementia. The transition from self-care to staff care can be marked by self-neglect if decline in function is not recognized early by nursing home staff or physicians.

Pressure ulcers are a common occurrence in the nursing home setting, which helps illustrate the complications surrounding elder abuse and neglect, particularly of dementia patients. Pressure ulcers are localized areas of soft-tissue injury resulting from compression of bony prominences and external surfaces. Four stages of pressure ulcers have been defined, ranging from nonblanchable erythema with intact skin (stage 1) to full-thickness skin loss with damage to the surrounding structures (stage 4). Seventeen percent to 35% of patients have been found in several studies to have pressure ulcers upon admission the nursing homes [48]. Pressure ulcer development among nursing home residents increase with the length of stay in a facility, with more than 20% of residents developing a pressure ulcer after 2 years in a nursing home [49]. Pressure ulcers have been the focus of much elder negligence litigation [50]. Traditionally, pressure ulcers have been attributed to poor nursing care. However, significant emphasis has been placed on pressure ulcer prevention strategies: a review of the literature found little change in the incidence of pressure ulcers [51].

Community and nursing home settings

There are multiple issues surrounding the abuse and neglect of persons with dementia, regardless of whether they are residing in the community or in nursing homes. In both settings, there are some similar characteristics that contribute to the potential for abuse and neglect. Patients at home and in nursing homes have care needs that may exceed the capabilities and time constraints of the caregivers. Caregivers at home may be juggling financial concerns, their own ailing health, children, and jobs with care of the elder. Even the most well-intentioned caregiver at home or in the nursing home has a finite amount of time to care for the patient. Low staff-to-patient ratios in the institutional setting, a common discrepancy, increase staff burden of care. In both settings, as patients' dementia progresses and their behavioral symptoms worsen, their need for care increases, and therefore the burden on the caregiver increases. Patients in either setting who exhibit aggressive behavior toward their caregivers are at greater risk of being physically or psychologically abused, whether it is as a reflex, in self-defense, or in response to frustration.

There are notable differences between dementia patients at home and in an institutional setting with respect to elder abuse. At a nursing home, patients are cared for by rotating nurses and nursing assistants, which creates a large pool of potential abusers but also a system of accountability and regulation. In the community, caregivers generally come from a small, intimate group of family and friends and may be hired caregivers. There is potentially more emotional investment in the care of the patient but less supervision. Education of caregivers is a key component of successful care of the dementia patient. In a nursing home, staff members undergo mandatory training on how to properly care for their patients. Although training is often provided on the mechanics of providing care, staff is usually not trained in ways to handle difficult interpersonal issues that arise with patients [47]. In the home setting, caregivers have varying degrees of awareness of their patients' needs. For example, well-intentioned caregivers may provide patients with improper amounts of food and water simply because they do not know the appropriate quantities, or patients may be restrained to "protect" them from wandering and falling.

Because of the research challenges associated with studying patients with cognitive impairments, the data available on elder abuse in nursing homes and in the home setting are limited. Definitions of abuse and neglect vary widely from state to state, and studies use different inclusion and exclusion criteria. In addition, in the nursing home setting, it is often difficult to distinguish abuse from bad practice or substandard care, which is also a serious concern but might be addressed differently. Obtaining a representative sample from the community or the nursing home pool poses a substantial challenge. In the community, studies are susceptible to the self-selection of survey participants. Nursing home facilities range widely with respect to size, services offered, patient populations, and other factors that could potentially influence study data [39,46].

Diagnosis of elder abuse in dementia patients

Recognizing elder abuse can be difficult. The American Medical Association has recommended that all older adults be asked by physicians about family violence even in the absence of overt symptoms that are suspicious for abuse or neglect because asymptomatic family violence often goes unrecognized [52]. Evaluations for suspected abuse should be thorough and may span several clinic visits. In the dementia patient, the diagnostic challenge may be increased by the elder's inability to recognize and report abusive behavior due to his cognitive deficits. In addition, the technique of interviewing the patient and suspected abuser separately to look for disparities is difficult due to the cognitive and memory impairments of the dementia patient. Therefore, corroborative information supplied by sources other than the caregiver and collected at a home visit may assist in making the diagnosis [21,53]. Empathy and understanding of caregiver burden should be emphasized as a nonjudgmental approach that generally yields more information than confrontation [17].

A history of behavior changes may be warning signs for elder abuse in dementia patients. Symptoms such as pseudo-seizures, elective mutism, aggressive behavior, refusal of medications, withdrawal, and limited eye contact may warrant further evaluation of possible abuse. Changes in appetite (eg, refusal to eat) or changes in sleep (eg, daytime sleep instead of night-time sleep or refusal to sleep alone) may be possible indications of abuse [54]. Historic findings of frequent admissions to multiple hospitals, surgeries secondary to trauma, and irregular medical follow-up raise suspicion of abuse [20]. In patients with adequate resources and a designated provider of care, inattention to established medical needs (eg, missed appointments or unfilled prescriptions) may reflect abuse or neglect [17].

The physical examination may yield crucial information toward an evaluation of elder abuse and neglect. In a review of emergency department records of elder abuse, the most common physical injuries among abused elders were unexplained bruises, lacerations, abrasions, head injury, and unexplained fractures [55]. Although dramatic cases of physical abuse are generally easily recognizable, most physical signs of elder abuse are more subtle. The diagnosis of severe neglect should be considered whenever a dependent patient with adequate resources and a designated provider of care presents with gross inattention to nutrition or hygiene [17]. Dehydration and malnutrition presented more commonly than injury among abused elders in the emergency room [55].

Many of the dementia patients at risk for abuse suffer from multiple chronic diseases. Although the suspicion for abuse may be present, medical professionals may be hesitant to attach an incorrect label of abuse or neglect. It is often difficult to distinguish the effects of the chronic disease and symptoms that could be expected as a natural course of the diseases from results of neglect and abuse. The behavioral changes mentioned previously may result from the progression of dementia. Frail elders sustain injuries easily and may self-injure as a result of disability [54]. Injuries that suggest abuse may occur spontaneously. For example, in one series of case reports, six nonweight-bearing elders were found with spontaneous long-bone fractures and no evidence of physical abuse, four of whom were reported for suspected abuse [56]. On the other hand, signs of abuse and neglect may often be wrongfully attributed to normal aging or degenerative processes. For example, hip fractures resulting from family violence may be erroneously ascribed to a common injury among elders with osteoporosis [17]. When physicians evaluate these elderly patients, they often focus on treating the immediate physical symptoms and ignore the potential implications of abuse [39].

Treatment, intervention, and prevention

Because management of elder abuse in dementia patients is complicated, efforts to address the problem must be taken on multiple fronts. Medical treatment of elder abuse focuses on the safety of the abuse victim. If the abuse is immediately threatening, treatment may include emergency removal from the site of abuse [17,52]. Attentive medical management, including hospitalization, is appropriate to treat the injuries sustained from physical abuse or neglect [17]. Goals of medical care should include interventions to maintain the patient's independence [27] and treatment of his or her aggressive behavior [22] to minimize risk factors for the onset of abuse.

Treatment and prevention of elder abuse should follow a multidisciplinary model. Regardless of the assessment technique used or intervention taken, elder abuse prevention requires health care provider follow-up and referral to appropriate resources in a multidisciplinary setting. Frequent interface with multiple agencies is thought to result in a higher rate of elder abuse reporting [57]. Anetzberger et al [58] have proposed a model intervention for elder abuse and dementia. In this model, they aim to increase case identification, improve care planning and intervention, and promote prevention of elder abuse in dementia patients. An educational curriculum on issues of abuse and dementia, a handbook for caregivers, a cross-training program for Alzheimer's Association and Adult Protective Services staff and volunteers, and a screening tool have been developed for this purpose.

A preventive approach to potentially abusive situations regarding elderly patients with and without dementia is repeatedly emphasized in elder abuse literature. Particularly with dementia patients, attention should be focused toward caregivers because caregivers are often the perpetrators of abuse. For example, interventions that enhance social support for the caregiver, including individual and family counseling, potentially alleviate abuse stemming from caregiver depression diagnosed by the Geriatric Depression Scale, which is a risk factor for abuse [22,32,59,60]. Support networks for caregivers with members with caregiving experience, especially status similar networks, have been shown to decrease violent feelings [61]. Assessing the level of caregiver burden through the Zarit Burden Interview (Box 1) and referring to respite care, support groups, and resources of education about the care recipient's disease and caregiving coping strategies are also recommended interventions [59]. Further, counseling the caregiver regarding the use of distracting and diversionary tactics with combative patients, maintaining routines and setting limits with the patient is beneficial to the health of the care dyad [22,60]. Addressing substance abuse and mood disorders on the part of either party may defuse a potentially abusive circumstance.

Health care personnel should be central in the management of elder abuse in dementia patients. If risk factors for abuse are identified, the health care provider has the opportunity to intervene to prevent abuse. The success of primary prevention of elder abuse rests on the ability of the health care provider to make assessments and interventions and to maintain a consistent relationship with patients and caregivers. The provider must reassess the level of caregiver burden and depression, which are risk factors for abuse [22,24,30,31,33].

Relative inattention of the medical and lay community to the prevalence of elder abuse is echoed in multiple reviews and is often attributed to discomfort with addressing the subject [20,31,52]. Education and training of providers and the general public to be aware of the problem of elder abuse is fundamental to the success of controlling it [57]. Clinicians may fail to report abuse due to underrecognition of or lack of information about the entity, ageism, lack of knowledge of reporting requirements and procedures, lack of confidence in public agencies to respond to reports, or protection of the physician-patient relationship

Box 1. The Zarit Burden Interview

Each question is scored between 0 (never) to 5 (nearly always). Higher total score indicates higher caregiver burden.

1. Do you feel that your relative asks for more help than he/she needs?
2. Do you feel that because of the time you spend with your relative that you don't have enough time for yourself?
3. Do you feel stressed between caring for your relative and trying to meet other responsibilities for your family or work?
4. Do you feel embarrassed over your relative's behavior?
5. Do you feel angry when you are around your relative?
6. Do you feel that your relative currently affects your relationships with other family members or friends in a negative way?
7. Are you afraid what the future holds for your relative?
8. Do you feel your relative is dependent on you?
9. Do you feel strained when you are around your relative?
10. Do you feel your health has suffered because of your involvement with your relative?
11. Do you feel that you don't have as much privacy as you would like because of your relative?
12. Do you feel that your social life has suffered because you are caring for your relative?
13. Do you feel uncomfortable about having friends over because of your relative?
14. Do you feel that your relative seems to expect you to take care of him/her as if you were the only one he/she could depend on?
15. Do you feel that you don't have enough money to take care of your relative in addition to the rest of your expenses?
16. Do you feel that you will be unable to take care of your relative much longer?
17. Do you feel you have lost control of your life since your relative's illness?
18. Do you wish you could leave the care of your relative to someone else?
19. Do you feel uncertain about what to do about your relative?
20. Do you feel you should be doing more for your relative?
21. Do you feel you could do a better job in caring for your relative?
22. Overall, how burdened do you feel in caring for your relative?

Adapted from Zarit Burden Interview, © Steven H. Zarit, 1983; with permission.

[29,57,62]. Training of health care personnel in psychiatry, public health and community medicine courses, and inclusion of elder abuse material in the curricula of emergency medicine, psychiatry, family medicine, and gynecology rotations are proposed measure to improve recognition and reporting of elder abuse [52]. The use of standardized assessment procedures for the assessment of elder abuse, such as a fixed intake form, has been suggested [20,21]. AMA guidelines advocate abuse and neglect screening for all elderly patients seen in a health care setting [63]. Self-education of physicians regarding related laws, legislation, and channels of reporting is encouraged. The health care provider is obligated in most states to report suspected abuse to a local governmental agency [52]. The Elder Abuse and Neglect Act specifies which service providers are responsible for reporting elder abuse [64].

Elder abuse intervention can be controversial with dementia patients, particularly in the setting of "unreasonable intrusion" of patient privacy and in the determination of when a person is too impaired cognitively to make his or her own decisions [35]. Health care providers are obligated to adhere to the ethical principles of autonomy, justice, beneficence, and nonmaleficence [20]. Applied to the cognitively intact elder, adherence to these principles may result in perpetuation of the abusive situation if the elder declines intervention despite the efforts and intentions of the clinician. Early in the course of dementia, decisional capacity may be difficult to judge. Therefore, the clinician may be conflicted in his or her obligations to respect patient autonomy and advocate for patient welfare. Furthermore, the principle of justice, intended to give each patient his or her rightful dues, may argue for removal of the patient unaware of his or her rights to a safe, un-exploited living environment.

Summary

Because of the impairments consequent to dementia, a unique relationship exists between dementia and elder abuse. Dementia has been controversially cited as a risk factor for elder abuse. This hypothesis is supported by the idea that disruptive symptoms, impairments, and dependencies associated particularly with late-stage dementia incite abusive behavior. Multiple other risk factors for abuse, such as caregiver stress, have been identified in community settings and in long-term care settings. Health care personnel are generally not aware of the special vulnerabilities of the dementia patient and fail to recognize elder abuse. Therefore, a first step in addressing the problem of elder abuse is to educate clinicians about the risk factors for elder abuse and to have a high index of suspicion for abuse in dementia patients. Education of caregivers regarding the clinical course of dementia and the anticipated needs of the care recipient is critical to successful care of the dementia patient and preemption of abuse precipitants. Support of caregivers, including treatment of caregiver depression and referral to community resources, may help prevent or stop abuse.

References

[1] Cummings JL, Arsland D, Jarvik L. Dementia. In: Cassel CK, Cohen HJ, Larson EB, et al, editors. Geriatric medicine. 3rd edition. New York: Springer Verlag; 1997.

[2] Cummings JL. Alzheimer's disease. N Engl J Med 2004;351:56–67.

[3] Hebert LE, Scherr PA, Bienias JL, et al. Alzheimer disease in the US population: prevalence estimates using the 2000 census. Arch Neurol 2003;60:1119–22.

[4] Evans DA, Funkenstein HH, Albert MS, et al. Prevalence of Alzheimer's disease in a community population of older persons: Higher than previously reported. JAMA 1989;262:2551–6.

[5] Kukull WA, Ganguli M. Epidemiology of dementia: concepts and overview. Neurol Clin 2000; 18:923–50.

[6] Bachman DL, Wolf PA, Linn RT, et al. Incidence of dementia and probable AD in a general population: the Framingham Study. Neurology 1993;43:515–9.

[7] Matthews FE, Dening T. Prevalence of dementia in institutional care. Lancet 2002;360:225–6.

[8] Messinger-Rapport BJ. Does this patient have Alzheimer disease? Diagnosing and treating dementia. Cleaveland Clin J Med 2003;70:762–76.

[9] Geldmacher DS, Whitehouse PJ. Evaluation of dementia. New Engl J Med 1996;335:330–6.

[10] Katzman R, Jackson JE. Alzheimer's disease: basic and clinical advances. J Am Geriatr Soc 1991;39:516–25.

[11] Teri L, Gibbons LE, McCurry SM. Exercise plus behavioral management in patients with Alzheimer disease: a randomized controlled trial. JAMA 2003;290:2015–22.

[12] Farlow MR. NMDA receptor antagonists: a new therapeutic approach for Alzheimer's disease. Geriatrics 2004;59:22–7.

[13] Tinetti ME, Liu W, Marattoli RA, et al. Mechanical restraint use among residents of skilled nursing facilities: prevalence, patterns, and predictors. JAMA 1991;265:468–71.

[14] Hayley DC, Cassel CK, Snyder L, et al. Ethical and legal issues. In: Medical care of the nursing home resident: what physicians need to know. Philadelphia: American College of Physicians; 1996. p. 143–54.

[15] Siegler EL, Capezuti E, Maislin G, et al. Effects of a restraint reduction intervention and OBRA '87 regulations on psychoactive drug use in nursing homes. J Am Geriatr Soc 1997;45: 791–6.

[16] Pillemer K, Finkelhor D. The prevalence of elder abuse: a random sample survey. Gerontologist 1988;28:51–7.

[17] Lachs MS, Pillemer K. Abuse and neglect of elderly persons. N Engl J Med 1995;332:437–43.

[18] The National Elder Abuse Incidence Study: final report. Washington, DC: Administration on Aging; 1998.

[19] Wolf R. Elder abuse and neglect: causes and consequences. J Geriatr Psychiatry 1997;30:153–74.

[20] Benton D, Marshall C. Elder abuse. Clin Geriatr Med 1991;7:831–45.

[21] Lachs MS, Fulmer T. Recognizing elder abuse and neglect. Geriatr Emerg Care 1993;9:665–75.

[22] Coyne AC, Reichman WE, Berbig LJ. The relationship between dementia and elder abuse. Am J Psychiatry 1993;150:643–6.

[23] Wolf RS. Caregiver stress, Alzheimer's Disease, and elder abuse. Am J Alzheimer Dis 1998; 2:81–3.

[24] Pavesa GJ, Cohen D, Eisdorfer C, et al. Severe family violence and Alzheimer's disease: prevalence and risk factors. Gerontologist 1992;32:493–7.

[25] Pillemer K, Finkelhor D. The prevalence of elder abuse: a random sample survey. Gerontologist 1988;28:51.

[26] Lachs MS, Williams C, O'Brien S, et al. Risk factors for reported elder abuse and neglect: a nine-year observational cohort study. Gerontologist 1997;37:469–74.

[27] Lachs MS, Berkman L, Fulmer T, et al. A prospective community-based pilot study of risk factors for the investigation of elder mistreatment. J Am Geriatr Soc 1994;42:169–73.

[28] Dyer CB, Pavlik VN, Murphy KP, et al. The high prevalence of depression and dementia in elder abuse and neglect. J Am Geriatr Soc 2000;48:205–8.

[29] Swagerty Jr DL, Takahashi PY, Evans JM. Elder mistreatment. Am Fam Physician 1999; 59:2804–8.
[30] Ory MG, Hoffman RR, Yee JL, et al. Prevalence and impact of caregiving: a detailed comparison between dementia and nondementia caregivers. Gerontologist 1999;39:177–85.
[31] Kleinschmidt KC. Elder abuse: a review. Ann Emerg Med 1997;30:463–72.
[32] Quayhagen M, Quayhagen MP, Patterson TL, et al. Coping with dementia: family caregiver burnout and abuse. J Mental Health Aging 1997;3:357–64.
[33] Mittelman MS, Ferris SH, et al. A comprehensive support program: effect on depression in spouse-caregivers of AD patients. Gerontologist 1995;35:792–802.
[34] Abrams RC, Lachs M, McAvay G, et al. Predictors of self-neglect in community-dwelling elders. Am J Psychiatry 2002;159:1724–30.
[35] Tueth MJ. Exposing financial exploitation of impaired elderly persons. Am J Geriatr Psychiatry 2000;8:104–11.
[36] Heisler CJ, Tewksbury JE. Fiduciary abuse of the elderly: a prosecutor's perspective. J Elder Abuse Neglect 1991;3:23–40.
[37] Hafemeister TL. Financial abuse of the elderly in domestic settings. In: Bonnie RJ, Wallace RB, editors. Elder mistreatment: abuse, neglect, and exploitation in an aging America. Washington, DC: National Academies Press; 2003. p. 382–445.
[38] Kemper P, Murtaugh CM. Lifetime use of nursing home care. N Engl J Med 1991;324:595–600.
[39] Hawes C. Elder abuse in residential long term care settings: what is known and what information is needed? In: Bonnie RJ, Wallace RB, editors. Elder mistreatment: abuse, neglect, and exploitation in an aging America. Washington, DC: National Academies Press; 2003. p. 446–500.
[40] Rubenstein LZ. Contexts of care. In: Cassel CK, Cohen HJ, Larson EB, et al, editors. Geriatric medicine. 3rd edition. New York: Springer Verlag; 1997.
[41] Galasko D, Corey-Bloom J, Thal LJ. Monitoring progression in Alzheimer's disease. J Am Geriatr Soc 1991;39:932–42.
[42] Spector WD, Fleishman JA, Pezzin LE, et al. Characteristics of long-term care users. Agency for healthcare research and quality, commissioned by Institute of Medicine, Committee on Improving Quality in Long-Term Care. Available at: www.ahrq.gov/research/ltcusers/. Accessed October 1, 2004.
[43] Besdine RW, Rubenstein LZ, Snyder L, editors. Medical care of the nursing home resident: what physicians need to know. Philadelphia: American College of Physicians; 1996.
[44] Pillemer K, Bachman-Prehn R. Helping and hurting: predictors of maltreatment of patients in nursing homes. Res Aging 1991;13:74–95.
[45] Monk A, Kaye LW, Litwin H. Resolving grievances in the nursing home: a study of the ombudsman program. New York: Columbia University Press; 1984.
[46] Nerenberg L. Abuse in nursing homes. Special research review section [newsletter]. Washington, DC: National Center on Elder Abuse; 2002.
[47] Pillemer K, Moore DW. Abuse of patients in nursing homes: findings from a survey of staff. Gerontologist 1989;29:314.
[48] Smith DM. Pressure ulcers in the nursing home. Ann Intern Med 1995;123:433–42.
[49] Brandeis GH, Morris JN, Nash DJ, et al. The epidemiology and natural history of pressure sores in elderly nursing home residents. JAMA 1990;264:2905–9.
[50] Bennett RG, O'Sullivan J, DeVito EM, et al. The increasing medical malpractice risk related to pressure ulcers in the United States. J Am Geriatr Soc 2000;48:73–81.
[51] Thomas DR. Are all pressure ulcers avoidable? J Am Med Dir Assoc 2001;2:297–301.
[52] Clarke ME, Wendell P. Management of elder abuse in the emergency department. Emerg Med Clin North Am 1999;17:631–44.
[53] Rubenstein LZ. The importance of including the home environment in assessment of frail older persons. J Am Geriatr Soc 1999;47:111–2.
[54] Baladerian NJ. Recognizing abuse and neglect in people with severe cognitive and/or communication impairments. J Elder Abuse Negl 1997;9:93–103.
[55] Jones J, Dougherty J, Shelble D, et al. Emergency department protocol for the diagnosis and evaluation of geriatric abuse. Ann Emerg Med 1988;17:1006–15.

[56] Kane RS, Goodwin JS. Spontaneous fractures of the long bones in nursing home patients. Am J Med 1991;90:263–6.

[57] Wolf RS, Li D. Factors affecting the rate of elder abuse reporting to a state protective services program. Gerontologist 1999;39:222–8.

[58] Anetzberger GJ, Palmisano BR, Sanders M, et al. A model intervention for elder abuse and dementia. Gerontologist 2000;49:492–7.

[59] Parks SM, Novielli KD. A practical guide to caring for caregivers. Am Family Physician 2000;62:2613–20.

[60] Silliman RA. Caregiving issues in the geriatric medical encounter. Clin Geriatr Med 2000; 16:51–60.

[61] Kilburn JC. Network effects in caregiver to care-recipient violence: a study of caregivers to those diagnosed with Alzheimer's Disease. J Elder Abuse Negl 1996;8:69–80.

[62] Sanders AB, Morley JE. The older person and the emergency department. J Am Geriatr Soc 1993;41:880–2.

[63] Aravanis SC, Adelman RD, Breckman R, et al. American Medical Association diagnostic and treatment guidelines on elder abuse and neglect. Chicago: American Medical Association; 1992.

[64] Blagojevich RR, Johnson CD. Elder abuse and neglect act and related laws including madated reporters and elder abuse provider agencies. Illinois Department on Aging, April 2003.

ELSEVIER
SAUNDERS

Clin Geriatr Med 21 (2005) 333–354

CLINICS IN
GERIATRIC
MEDICINE

Elder Abuse and Neglect in Long-Term Care

Seema Joshi, MD[a,*], Joseph H. Flaherty, MD[a,b]

[a]Geriatric Research, Education and Clinical Center, St. Louis VA Medical Center,
1402 South Grand Boulevard, Room M238, St. Louis, MO 63104, USA
[b]Division of Geriatrics, Department of Internal Medicine, Saint Louis University School of Medicine,
1402 South grand Boulevard, St. Louis, MO 63104, USA

Long-term care (LTC) can be defined based on the characteristics of the person receiving care. The most useful image of an older person who receives or needs LTC is of an older person who is frail, disabled, or has multiple chronic conditions. Whether one believes these conditions have so much overlap that it is difficult to distinguish them or whether one believes these are distinct clinical entities that are causally related and can improve our understanding and treatment of older persons [1], most health care professionals would agree that older persons with any or all three of these conditions comprise the vast majority of those who receive LTC.

LTC can also be defined by the site at which a person receives care. The two sites discussed are in this article nursing homes (NHs) and the home. Although most of the lay publicity about abuse and neglect comes from NHs, it is necessary to include the home as a site of LTC because of the increasing use of this location as a site where chronic care for older persons with frailty, disability, or multiple chronic conditions is provided by health care workers. These health care workers have similar backgrounds to caregivers in NHs (eg, nurses, nurse assistants, social workers, therapists), but they are often alone with the patient, which creates different circumstances than in the NH setting.

Some 1.6 million people reside in approximately 17,000 nursing homes [2]. Although this is only a fraction of the United States population over 65 years of age (approximately 5%) this figure is misleading [3]. Among those 65 to

This work was supported in part by the Bureau of Health Professions' Geriatric Academic Career Award 5 K01 HP 00007.

* Corresponding author.

E-mail address: joshis@slu.edu (S. Joshi).

74 years of age, the rate is less than 2%. It rises to approximately 7% for those 75 to 84 years of age and jumps to 20% for those 85 and older. The proportion of people spending time in the nursing home is likely to increase if NHs continue to play a role in subacute care. In 1997, 15% of hospital patients 65 years of age or older were discharged to nursing homes. Compared with those going home or to rehabilitation units, older persons admitted to NHs are likely to have worse functional status and more confusion [3], which are potential risk factors for abuse and neglect.

Through the late 1990s, home care was the fastest growing segment of the Medicare budget, with expenditures increasing at a rate of 20% per year [4]. There are many reasons for this, but one of the main reasons is the growing population over the age of 85. It is unknown what percentage of people over 85 require home care services, but if only 20% are in NHs, a large percentage are still at home, many of whom have chronic illnesses.

Definitions

Past research demonstrates that consistent definitions of elder abuse are difficult to obtain [5]. Fulmer and O'Malley [6] define elder abuse as "actions of a caretaker that create unmet needs for elderly persons" and define neglect as "the failure of an individual responsible for caretaking to respond adequately to established needs for care." Another definition of elder abuse suggests that elder abuse is a category of elder mistreatment. Elder mistreatment is defined as "self or other inflicted suffering unnecessary to the maintenance of quality of life of the older person and identified as one or more behavioral manifestations, categorized as physical, psychological, sociologic, or legal circumstances"[7]. Some authors suggest that because one of the hallmarks of prevention of abuse and neglect is awareness, descriptions of patterns and even anecdotal stories are useful educational tools: "the CNA's (Certified Nurse Assistant) would first stop range of motion exercises, then stop helping residents eat, and third, stop maintaining hydration. Cries for water were one of the most common requests heard from residents" [8].

The definitional problem is complicated by the fact that there are 50 states dealing with the mistreatment of older persons, each of which uses its own set of definitions. The National Aging Resource Center on Elder Abuse has suggested defining institutional elder abuse as "all forms of maltreatment of older people (60 or 65 years of age and older depending on the state program) that takes place in institutional settings (instead of domestic or home setting)" [9]. This definition is too broad to be useful if the purpose of defining something is an effort to more clearly identify it and subsequently prevent it. A more practical approach may be to look at the various forms it can take (eg, physical, psychologic, sexual, medication, spiritual, financial, material, neglect, or socioeconomic).

We offer two approaches to defining elder abuse and neglect in LTC. The first is a definition based on the various forms abuse and neglect can take. It is the one used by the Office of the Inspector General of the Department of Health & Human Services and the one that we refer to during most of this article.

Forms of abuse and neglect

The Office of the Inspector General of the Department of Health & Human Services has identified seven different types of elder abuse of nursing home residents: physical abuse, misuse of restraints, verbal/emotional abuse, physical neglect, medical neglect, verbal/emotional neglect, and personal property abuse (material goods) [9].

Physical abuse is defined as the infliction of physical pain or injury. It includes sexual abuse. Examples include individuals reacting inappropriately to a situation, such as pushing or slapping a resident, or intentionally doing bodily harm.

Misuse of restraints includes chemical or physical control of a resident beyond physician's orders or not in accordance with accepted medical practice. Examples include staff failing to loosen the restraints within adequate time frames or attempting to cope with a resident's behavior by the inappropriate use of drugs.

Verbal or emotional abuse is defined as infliction of mental or emotional suffering. Examples include demeaning statements, harassment, threats, humiliation, or intimidation of the resident.

Physical neglect is defined as disregard for necessities of daily living. Examples include failure to provide necessary food, clothing, clean linens, or daily care of the resident's necessities (eg, brushing a resident's hair, helping with a resident's bath).

Medical neglect consists of lack of care for existing medical problems. Examples include ignoring a necessary special diet, not calling a physician when necessary, not being aware of the possible negative effects of medications, or not taking action on a medical problem.

Verbal or emotional neglect means creating situations in which esteem is not fostered. Examples include not considering a resident's wishes; restricting contact with family, friends, or other residents; or ignoring a resident's need for verbal and emotional contact.

Personal property abuse (material goods) is defined as the illegal or improper use of a resident's property by another for personal gain. Examples include the theft of a resident's private television, false teeth, clothing, or jewelry.

Definition based on interviews of nurses in nursing homes

The second approach to defining elder abuse and neglect is offered in a qualitative study by Hirst that involved interviews of nurses in a nursing home [10]. Hirst emphasized that researchers and governmental officials have used definitions developed outside LTC facilities to define elder abuse and neglect in institutional settings. These definitions may not convey the meaning of the term as it is used internally by staff and residents within the facility [11]. This approach may have more potential than the first approach to help caregivers, researchers, and policy makers understand the nature of why elder abuse and neglect occurs in LTC and thus may help with prevention. This study is limited by the fact that nurse's aides were not included in the study.

Ten registered nurses from five nursing homes were interviewed to determine their perception of resident abuse. The study tried to define resident abuse as it is used by registered nurses within long-term care institutions. The description that the study participants gave assisted in defining resident abuse into the following five categories: (1) perception of hurt, (2) commission or omission, (3) context of care, (4) intentional or unintentional act, and (5) behavioral clusters.

Perception of hurt

Nurses defined a behavior as resident abuse if it produced a perception of hurt in an older resident. Abuse means there is hurt that the resident feels physically or emotionally. Some residents are able to verbalize their perception of hurt and for others; their physical conditions make it impossible for them to express their hurt. In the case of the latter, the nurses made the decision of abuse on their behalf.

Commission or omission

Commission describes performed behaviors; something you do, such as deciding not to get the resident's hearing aid, shoving the resident into the chair, or removing personal items without the resident's permission. Omission describes actions left undone. As described by one of the nurses, "there is so much to do, so you can't do it all and you leave some things undone."

Context of care

Nurses placed behavior ascribed to resident abuse within a context of care framework. Context is defined as the circumstance and the environment in which the experience of abuse occurred. Context is differentiated into two subcategories: context bound and context free. Context bound means that the environment always influences the perception of an experience as resident abuse. For example, the use of restraints is influenced by the nurses' perception of the need for them; if a need is perceived then their use is not considered resident abuse. Context free means that an act is resident abuse regardless of the circumstance in which it occurred (eg, pinching, hitting, or gripping too hard).

Intentional or unintentional act

The acts of resident abuse could be intentional or unintentional. The criterion used to differentiate between the two is the reason behind the act. When the goal is to hurt, the behavior is resident abuse. For example, a nonprofessional staff wanted to hurt a resident—perhaps teach her a lesson. The resident had bitten her, and she bit the resident back. Unintentional does not have as its goal the causing of hurt. As one nurse said, "I was moving her up in bed and she said that I hurt her but I didn't mean to." Another example is of a resident who fractured her hip because the personal care aide did not want to wait for the lift to be free; she did not mean to do it, but she did.

Behavioral clusters

Abusive actions were grouped into behavioral clusters. There are five clusters of intentional acts: offensive language, physical acts, material acts, failure to meet physical needs, and failure to meet psychosocial needs. Unintentional acts are divided into clusters of inappropriate language, failure to meet physical needs, and failure to meet psychosocial needs. Examples include using the words "bib" or "diapers," which are inappropriate and degrading. Forgetting that a patient with Alzheimer disease can feel pain demonstrates failure to meet physical needs. An example of the failure to meet psychosocial needs is taking a resident to the lounge for the piano player just because the staff decides that it is good for her.

Scope of the problem

Evidence of existence and the data on prevalence of elder abuse and neglect in LTC settings comes from numerous sources including media, incidents drawn from anecdotal cases in LTC facilities reported to governmental agencies for investigation, analysis of databases of state nursing home inspections, surveys of staff, and research studies. The issue of abuse and neglect in LTC facilities has appeared in several newspapers and magazines. Examples include a single case in Virginia concerning abuse in a nursing home, use of physical and chemical restraints in California along with stories from victims and their families recounting institutional abuse, and an anecdotal account of one woman's experience with death of her father due to alleged abuse and neglect in the nursing home [12–14].

In 1995, more than 300 confirmed cases of abuse or neglect were reported by Virginia, Maryland, and District of Columbia nursing homes [9]. Nationwide, over 1.6 million people reside in nursing homes. Although these kinds of reports highlight the seriousness of the problem, they cannot be used to calculate the true incidence of the problem. A government report, prepared by the Special Investigations Division of the House Government Reform Committee in 2001, found that 30% of nursing homes in the United States, which represented approximately 5200 out of 17,000 homes, were cited for almost 9000 abuse violations during 1999 and 2000. The abuse consisted of physical, sexual, verbal, and other abuse. More than 1600 nursing homes were cited for violations that caused "actual harm to residents" or "placed the residents in immediate jeopardy of death or serious injury" [15].

A random sample of 577 nurses and nurses aides working in 32 NHs were asked about their observations concerning physical and psychologic abuse in the past year. Overall, 21% of the group observed excessive use of restraints, 17% observed "pushing, grabbing, shoving or pinching," and 12% observed "slapping or hitting." Six percent of the staff admitted to using restraints excessively; 3% admitted to "pushing, grabbing, shoving, or pinching" residents; and 3% had "slapped or hit" a resident. Observation of and committing acts of psychologic abuse was higher. Seventy percent had observed others yelling at patients in anger, and 33% had done yelled at patients. Fifty percent had observed others insulting or swearing at patients, and 10% had done this [16]. In a survey of 80 residents who lived in a nursing home (none had dementia) in 23 nursing homes, 44% said they had been physically abused, and 48% said they had been treated roughly (eg, flung into bed, shoved, and jerked). The details of how these 80 residents were recruited were not available, but these data suggest a difference between nursing and resident perception of the problem [8].

Using data from the Minimum Data Set for home care on 701 individuals 60 years of age and older in Michigan, researchers found a prevalence of potential elder abuse of 4.7% [17]. Although there is a paucity of other prevalence data for home care, research on elder abuse in the domestic setting suggests that elder abuse occurs 2% to 4% of the elderly population. The National Aging Resource Center on Elder Abuse speculates that for every report of elder abuse taken, there are 14 unreported cases [18].

A separate comment about sexual abuse is necessary. Analysis of data from 20 NH residents who were raped revealed several important findings that dispel myths and stereotypes. The study noted that (1) someone other than the victim reported the rape to an official; (2) unless a rape was witnessed, the report was delayed; (3) clues, such as a sexually transmitted disease, assisted in the disclosure of a rape; (4) victims' ability to communicate was impaired; (5) offenders were NH employees or other residents; and (6) physical and forensic evidence was missing if the examination was delayed [19].

The economic costs of abuse range from investigation procedures, health care interventions, and law enforcement activities to the lost productivity of those involved in the experience. These costs fall on society. The personal costs range from loss of dignity and personhood to physical trauma and perhaps early death [10].

Risk factors

The purpose of identifying risk factors associated with elder abuse and neglect is to raise awareness among caregivers of certain patient populations and to help focus interventions depending on which factors are present within particular sites of care. Within NHs, risk factors can be present among the residents of the NH or the staff. Within home care, risk factors may be identified among patients, family caregivers, or home care workers. Careful questioning and assessment can help determine whether a patient is at increased risk [20].

Various factors have been suggested from studies of cases in domestic settings [21] A 9-year observational cohort study has identified several risk factors in community-dwelling individuals [22]. These studies and studies from NHs and home care were evaluated to develop the following list of risk factors.

Patient characteristics

Age and gender

Although one study using data derived from the Medicaid Fraud Unit found that only 4% of the victims were under the age of 59 years [21], it cannot be concluded that older age is a risk factor because the majority of NH residents and home care patients are older than 59 years. In one home care study, age was not associated with potential abuse [17]. Male gender may be a risk factor because one study found that 56.7% of victims of elder abuse were men [21], although the proportion of women in NHs is higher than men. The study of home care patients did not find an association with gender [17].

Dementia or cognitive decline

Persons in NHs with dementia or cognitive decline are at an increased risk for abuse and neglect [8]. The mere presence of cognitive or functional impairment is not nearly as compelling a risk factor for mistreatment as the trajectory of decline [22]. Among home care patients, one study showed that dementia was not associated with potential abuse, whereas short-term memory loss and any psychiatric diagnosis were [17]. Another study of caregivers of cognitively impaired family members showed a relationship between mild dementia and abuse [23].

Disturbing behavior and poor conflict tactics

Disturbing behavior and poor conflict tactics may predispose to abuse [6]. Disruptive or insulting behavior by the older adult may be a factor because resident behaviors can be provocative [24]. Severely confused and aggressive residents were found to be often denied opportunities for personal choices in bathing, dressing, and eating; were isolated more often; and were left alone for long periods and labeled as "bad" with no effort to discover what prompted the aggressive behavior [25,26]. Patients with dementia often exhibit behavioral problems during the course of the dementia, but the behaviors described here can be seen among NH residents and home care patients without dementia [27].

Physical dependency or impairment of activities of daily living

Physical dependency or impairment of activities of daily living (ADLs) is considered a factor in the interpersonal dynamics between victim and abuser [20]. According to one review of the literature, one of the best predictors for unintentional weight loss among NH residents, once terminal illness is excluded, is the need for help with eating. Approximately a quarter of residents of assisted living facilities who reported needing help with toileting did not receive that help. Physically or mentally frail elderly persons were found to receive less humane and respectful treatment from staff because they demonstrated greater dependence and were more difficult for staff to relate to as people [25,28]. Impaired ADLs was not associated with potential abuse among home care patients according to one study [17].

Staff risk factors

Gender

Studies on the impact of gender on elder abuse have revealed that male employees were more likely to abuse male residents and that female employees are more likely to abuse female residents. Analysis in one study revealed 62.9% of the incidents of elder abuse involved a male employee. The fact that more men are accused of abuse was surprising because traditionally more women have been employed in the nursing home industry [21].

Caregiver burden

Caregiver burden is a well-recognized problem in NHs. In one study, a nurses' aide reported that when staff became overtired and overwhelmed, their response to a resident who causes trouble is often aggressive. Five main sources of stress for nurses' aides were identified in one study: residents, bureaucratic rules, supervisors who valued efficiency over compassion and failed to provide role models, family relationships (the worker's family and resident's family), and coworkers [29].

Ageism

In one study, about 75% of the NH staff believed that dementia, confusion, anger, and incontinence were a normal part of aging. Although this may qualify as ageism, the intent by labeling this risk factor as such is not to judge, keeping in mind that ageism is found in numerous other sites of health care [30–32]. The intent is to help figure out why these beliefs occur. Why is it that nurses' aides comprise the largest group of those accused of elder abuse? This may be due to the sheer numbers of nurses' aides and the amount of time they spend with the patients. However, it is plausible that an inadequate level or type of training might contribute to this finding [21].

Staff burnout and poor/short staffing

Burnout among nurses and nurses' aides is a factor with profound implications for institutional elder abuse. Burnout is characterized by progressive physical and emotional exhaustion involving the development of negative job attitudes and perception [33]. Although staff/patient ratios have been less studied than the issue of burnout, workload demands are implicated as a risk factor for elder abuse and neglect in NHs [34]. These factors have not been well studied in home care.

Risk factors among home care workers have not been fully elucidated, but one study suggests that at least the model of care—agency-based care compared with consumer-directed care—did not make a difference concerning abuse risk [35]. Although there are no studies comparing attitudes of nurses in NHs and home care, nurses may view older persons in their own home as more autonomous and independent [36] and may view themselves as having more time and less stress when dealing with patients in a one-on-one environment [37].

Criminal record

Although this has not been looked at in studies related to elder abuse and neglect, criminal record should be considered a risk factor among staff in NHs and especially in home care.

Facility characteristics

The ownership status of a facility (whether for-profit or nonprofit institution) may be related to maltreatment. Recent research suggests that nonprofit homes are superior medical and personal care facilities. Rates charged by the facility have been found to be associated with better institutional quality [38]. Although NHs charging higher rates might seem to have lower rates of maltreatment because they can hire more staff with better training [38], one study did not find an association between lower charge rates or for-profit status and physical or psychologic abuse rates [16].

Family caregiver characteristics

Caregiver personality problems

Although the burden and stress related to caring for family members who are ill and dependent would seem to be a major risk factor for abuse and neglect, one study found more support for the idea that abuse is associated with personality problems of the caregiver [39]. These problems were described as "abuser deviance" and included destroying property, having hit someone else, having been arrested, psychiatric problems, alcohol and drug problems, and physical health problems.

Clues for suspecting elder abuse and neglect

A comprehensive geriatric assessment, including social and financial information, is a good tool for gathering clues that may raise suspicion of abuse and neglect [40]. We review physical findings that may raise suspicion that is especially pertinent to NH residents but that could apply to home care patients. Although the physical examination may provide important clues for differentiating abuse and neglect from disease or age-related physiologic changes [20], a positive physical finding does not always mean that abuse or neglect has occurred. Thus, when one of these findings is present, an immediate judgment that abuse or neglect has occurred is not warranted. Further evaluation (eg, more history from all involved parties and consideration of other reasons for the findings) is the next step.

Using the Office of the Inspector General definitions for different types of abuse, we have categorized physical findings into those that may raise suspicion for physical abuse and those that raise suspicion for physical or medical neglect, with cautions in each category about differentiating abuse and neglect from illness, disease, or age-related changes.

Physical abuse

Bruises or skin tears

Although these can be signs of physical abuse, easy bruising can occur in patients on various types of medications. Medications such as aspirin, warfarin, and clopidogrel can cause bleeding and may produce ecchymosis. Simple trauma may result in a skin tear because there is reduced contact between epidermis and dermis with age, which results in an epidermis that separates easily from the dermis. There may also be a decrease in the number of cutaneous nerves, which reduces sensitivity to touch and pain, making elderly persons more susceptible to burns [41].

As use of complementary and alternative therapies continues to rise in the United States [42] and as use of these therapies is seen among older patients [43], health care workers need to be aware of certain techniques, such as cupping and moxibustion, that may mimic physical abuse [44].

Multiple fractures/long bone fractures

Osteoporosis increases with age, as do falls and metastatic cancer, all of which increase the risk for fractures and thereby increase the chance that physical abuse will result in fractures. Thus, if physical abuse is suspected, physicians may consider doing radiographic studies that are not typically done, such as radiographs of ribs and small bones. Long-bone fracture may be a sign of physical abuse. However, spontaneous fractures of the long bones do occur in NH patients in the absence of trauma. Patients at risk for such fractures typically have been bedridden or nonweight bearing for several years [45]. In this study, there was no evidence of physical abuse in any of these patients; indeed, evidence against abuse was fairly good. It is important that this phenomenon be recognized to avoid unexplained fractures in NH patients being taken as evidence of abuse or neglect.

In addition to facial radiographs to evaluate for maxillofacial injuries, physicians should be aware of the occurrence of subdural hematomas as a result of physical abuse [46,47].

Pelvic findings

The forensic examination in case of rape can be challenging for many reasons. The patient may resist the pelvic examination because of injury or pain, and the pelvic area may be difficult to visualize because of leg contractures. Explaining the examination to a victim who has dementia or is cognitively impaired may be difficult. The primary evidence relating to a sexual assault is the presence of semen and bruising in the pelvic area. Secondary evidence includes vaginal or purulent discharge, evidence of a sexually transmitted disease, or positive findings of blood [48].

Physical or medical neglect

Unintended weight loss

Although one could consider that one of the causes of unintentional weight loss is physical or medical neglect, this explanation does not address the underlying causes of weight loss in the NH and does not help in preventing it from happening. For example, one study revealed that once terminal illness was excluded, the best predictor for unintended weight loss among nursing home residents was the need for help in eating. Another study showed that one of the most common causes of weight loss was depression, even if patients with cancer were included in the group [49]. Are these examples of physical neglect or medical neglect? Was it the nurses' fault the patients did not eat, or was the need to help in eating related to the apraxia of dementia, dental factors, or something as simple as an inappropriate "low salt, low cholesterol" diet? Is missing or not treating depression in NH residents medical neglect? Because of the complexity of this issue, instead of claiming neglect immediately, we recommend review and application of guidelines to address this issue [50].

Home care patients are also at risk of malnutrition [51]. Although many of the recommendations in the guidelines noted previously [50] may apply to older persons receiving home care, other options and ideas exist [52,53].

Poor basic hygiene, poor oral and dental hygiene

Findings related to these areas are complex. Although emergency health care staff and hospital staff are justified in considering neglect as a factor when older patients come from a NH or home with poor hygiene, they are obligated to obtain the whole story before judgment can be made. The following are some common reasons to think about when patients arrive in this condition: Has the patient been refusing to bathe? Has the patient's acute (or subacute) illness, particularly a lethargic type delirium, prevented them from doing their hygiene when before they had been doing this independently?

Health care workers should be familiar with Diogenes syndrome. This is characterized by what seems to be extreme self-neglect, related to the persons home environment. One of the first reports of 30 elderly persons thought to have had this syndrome showed that all had dirty, untidy homes and a filthy personal appearance about which they showed no shame. Hoarding of rubbish (syllogomania) was sometimes seen. Poverty and poor housing standards were not a serious problem. An acute presentation with falls or collapse was common, as were nutritional deficiency states including iron, folate, vitamin B12, vitamin C, calcium, vitamin D, serum proteins, albumin, and potassium [54]. Some more recent reviews are recommended [55,56].

Oral care is a challenge and can be time consuming [57]. Although dentists play an important role in oral care, much of what is needed can be done by nurses and nurses' aids. The major challenge is the time this takes. However, those who make decisions about staff/patient ratios need to know that oral care is worthwhile in NHs and the home care setting [58].

Dehydration

Although dehydration may raise suspicion for medical and physical neglect, this diagnosis should be used with caution because physicians in hospitals often overdiagnose this based on physical examination findings that are not dependable. In a meta-analysis, McGee et al [59] found that in patients (many of whom were older) with vomiting, diarrhea, or decreased oral intake, none of the typical findings of dry mucous membranes, dry tongue, furrowed tongue, and sunken eyes were helpful when present in isolation. An increasing number of these findings with confusion, extremity weakness, and nonfluent speech might be helpful, but the authors concluded that this needed further validation. Only the presence of a dry axilla supported the diagnosis of hypovolemia. Moist mucous membranes and a tongue without furrows argued against it. A study by Thomas et al [60] showed that physicians who diagnosed dehydration during hospital admission seemed to rely more on physical signs than on laboratory data. Furthermore, little change in laboratory markers for hydration status occurred from the time of diagnosis to hospital discharge, suggesting that the clinical diagnosis did not affect fluid management. The importance of this is twofold. Because this diagnosis is often made at transfer to a hospital from home or a NH, it is important to recognize the difficulty in accurately making this diagnosis lest all patients labeled with dehydration be considered neglected. Second, the diagnosis of dehydration is considered a sentinel event for NHs, and inappropriate use of this diagnosis can cause undue harm to NHs.

Pressure ulcers are perhaps one of the most obvious and dramatic physical findings that create suspicion for neglect [20] and have been one of the main reasons for increased regulatory oversight in NHs. The issue of pressure ulcers has raised awareness of neglect in NHs, but the issue has created some misperceptions of NHs and fear of litigation. Despite increased regulatory oversight and improvements in technologies available for prevention, epidemiologic data demonstrate stability in the incidence. The possible explanation for this stable incidence of pressure ulcers includes a failure of known effective preventive treatment to be applied or the failure of prevention strategies to be effective in spite of being applied. No intervention strategy has been reported that consistently and reproducibly eliminates the incidence of pressure ulcers, and the published data on prevention of pressure ulcers do not support an assumption that all pressure ulcers are preventable [61]. Thus, the presence of pressure ulcers should raise serious concern, but the determination that the pressure ulcers are due to neglect should be made carefully.

Home care patients can develop pressure ulcers. In a multisite study of 13 home care agencies with over 2800 patients, over one third of the patients had a wound of some sort, and one fourth of the wounds were pressure ulcers [62]. Interventions, sometimes unique to the home setting, exist to prevent and treat these [62,63].

Social isolation and withdrawal

Careful in-depth interviews and observations may uncover depression or learned passive behavior that indicates a resignation to the abusive behavior. Although these behaviors may be subtle, may be ones that physicians and health care workers do not typically screen for, and may be attributable to ageing, observations such as fearful actions, withdrawing to touch, edginess, or restlessness, especially when the possible abuser is present, should raise suspicions [18].

Barriers to reporting or investigating elder abuse and neglect

Everyone who comes into contact with the older person has this responsibility of reporting abuse and neglect of NH residents and patients receiving home care services. This only includes those who work in the NH and in the home and those outside the immediate realm of these sites (eg, volunteers [64], emergency department and emergency response personnel [65], and intensive care unit nurses [66]). It may seem impractical for all these people outside of the immediate sites to report suspicious cases to adult protective services (APS) at the risk of causing the APS to be overwhelmed. However, without reporting, there is no investigation, and without investigation, prejudice and misperception of these sites by health care workers outside these sites will continue.

Although all states have laws concerning reporting, as of 1996, 42 states had APS laws containing mandatory reporting requirements directed toward health care and social service professionals. There are several practical, ethical, and controversial issues around mandatory reporting that are beyond the scope of this article but are outlined in a review by Capezuti et al [67]. Ideal APS legislation should include immunity of reporters from civil and criminal liability, establish procedures for emergency orders of protection, support special services for victims, and include appropriation of adequate funds to sustain a quality APS system [67].

Barriers in the NH for reporting abuse and neglect include ageism and inadequate training of LTC institution staff. Staff may have prejudiced attitudes and beliefs that dementia, anger, and incontinence are a normal part of aging. In one analysis, of 27 geographic areas in Massachusetts served by protective agencies, higher rates of reporting elder abuse were associated with more community training of area professionals and higher agency service rating scores [68].

Fear of retaliation and belief that it would not help may stop residents of NHs and persons living at home from complaining or telling anyone about abuse or neglect. Lack of awareness among family members of a problem until it has existed for too long may impair proper reporting. A significant time delay in investigation may occur (maybe as long as 14 days), allowing accurate memory of an event to fade or that offending staff to leave the facility. Lack of sufficient evidence may be an important factor. If the facility cannot identify the perpetrator, especially if a patient with dementia has bruises and cannot say who caused them, the case may be closed.

Home care workers face unique challenges in the decision to report elder abuse and neglect. Because one of the goals of care in the home is to prevent institutionalization, one of the common fears of reporting abuse and neglect is that institutionalization will be the consequence. One study of 2812 community-dwelling older persons, a subset of who were referred to elder protective services over a 9-year follow-up period, bears this out [69]. Rates of nursing home placement were 69.2% for self-neglecting subjects, 52.3% for mistreated subjects, and 31.8% for subjects who had no contact with APS. Risk of placement due to APS referral for self-neglect and for elder mistreatment exceeded those for other medical, functional, and social factors. However, reporting may lead to an increase in needed services for the patient and the family [70,71].

Not knowing how to report or to whom to report should not be seen as a barrier. The Administration on Aging (AoA) sponsors an Eldercare Locator service (1-800-677-1116) that refers callers to local agencies to report abuse. The AoA has a web site with general information on elder abuse and neglect [72]. The National Center on Elder Abuse, funded by the AoA, is a nonprofit (but not federal) organization. Its web site provides a state-by-state listing of toll-free telephone numbers to call when reporting elder abuse, whether the site is the NH or the home [73].

Prevention

The Health Care Financing Administration has offered the following guidelines for abuse prevention [74].

- Screening of all potential employees for a history of abuse, neglect, or mistreatment should be done. A thorough background screening is a worthwhile measure in safeguarding the residents and staff.
- Training all employees in abuse prohibition from day of hire to retire is essential. Focus should be on caring for difficult residents and on em-

ployees who are experiencing stressful duties and are at risk for burnout. Staff must know what constitutes abuse, mistreatment, neglect, and misappropriation of resident property.

• Prevention is one of the most complex of the components of the guidelines. All nursing home residents and their family members must know how and where to report events that they believe are abusive or neglectful. Dynamic care planning and resident education is essential. Residents and stake-holders of the LTC process need to be involved.

• Identification involves vigilance by direct care staff to observe residents for signs of abuse (eg, bruising, mood change, withdrawal, distrust, and so forth); there should be vigilance by management staff to assure all suspected cases are reported.

• The regulations require that there should be procedures for investigating all types of incidents and reporting results to the proper authorities. Investigation of cases should be assigned to qualified and trained individuals.

• Protection of residents from harm during the investigation must be done. The proximate cause must be identified as quickly as possible and extinguished immediately.

• The prevention process hinges on reporting. All staff must be coached to know that reporting abuse is not bad. Forty-two states have mandatory reporting laws for even suspected abuse, and all states have some system for reporting abuse through adult protective services or through a state long-term care ombudsman program [75,76].

Interventions

Table 1 has a partial list of recommended interventions, depending on the type of risk factor present. These recommendations are based on a synthesis of the literature, and although they are not evidence based because of the lack of and unethical nature of randomized trials of persons at risk for abuse and neglect, they do offer targeted areas for health care workers, administrators, policy makers, and educators.

Table 1 can be used to target specific risk factors if a particular type of abuse or neglect is identified. For example, if theft of personal property has become a problem among home care patients or within a NH, then administration will know it might be necessary to be more aggressive about doing background checks [77]. Although there is some degree of overlap within categories and the related types of abuse and neglect are not all inclusive for every risk factor, the table does allow a more focused approach for a facility or home care agency when abuse or neglect occurs rather than institutional-wide changes that are more difficult to achieve.

Behavioral problems among NH residents and older persons receiving home care are most commonly seen among persons with dementia. Because nursing

Table 1
Overview of most important risk factors, related types of abuse or neglect, and recommended interventions for nursing homes and home care

Location	Risk factor	Related type of abuse or neglect	Recommended intervention
Nursing homes	Patient with behavioral problems	Physical abuse Misuse of restraints Verbal/emotional abuse Physical neglect Medical neglect Verbal/emotional neglect	Special training Special units Alternative NH models
	Staff caregiver burden	Physical abuse Misuse of restraints Verbal/emotional abuse Physical neglect Medical neglect Verbal/emotional neglect	Improve staff/resident ratios Volunteer programs Alternative NH models Background checks?
	Staff burnout	Verbal/emotional abuse Physical neglect Medical neglect Verbal/emotional neglect	Staff support techniques Training
	Staff ageism	Misuse of restraints Physical neglect Medical neglect	Education Ombudsman Review residents' rights
	Staff discipline problems	Physical abuse Misuse of restraints Personal property	Background checks
Home care	Caregiver (family) personality problems	Physical abuse Misuse of restraints Verbal/emotional abuse Physical neglect Medical neglect Verbal/emotional neglect Personal property	Educate home care workers about this risk factor; use of multidisciplinary team; reporting
	Home care worker characteristics	Medical neglect Personal property	Background checks
	Patient psychosocial problems (isolation, psychiatric illnesses poor social support, refuses help)	Physical neglect Medical neglect Verbal/emotional neglect	Focus on resources available and use of multidisciplinary team instead of "rescuing"

Abbreviation: NH, nursing home.

assistants spend the most time with these persons, they should be given priority for special training and education in this area [78–80].

A variety of special environments exist for persons with dementia [81–84]. Although special units are helpful, one group of authors suggests that the psychosocial environment is the most important element of institutional care for persons with dementia. They argue that an emphasis on the psychosocial aspect of the environment may improve disruptive behavior through preservation of personhood, simple recognition of remaining abilities, a decreased focus on disabilities, and reduction of pharmacologic therapy [85].

Alternative NH models of living arrangement for persons with dementia, even moderate to severe dementia, are emerging. The commonalities of at least two of these models include smaller numbers of residents and a more consistent, smaller number of "universal" health care workers [86,87].

Relief of staff caregiver burden and prevention of staff burnout are challenging issues for NHs. Although improving staff/resident ratios seems to be the most logical solution, at least in one study of over 570 nurses about their observations of abuse and neglect in NHs, the quality of staff-to-resident interactions seemed to be a stronger predictor of abuse than the structure of the NH [16]. Nonetheless, many NHs are understaffed, and proper ratios are an important part of quality care. A qualitative study of nursing assistants found that they deemed their relationships with residents to be the central determinant of quality of care, and adequate staffing was essential to allowing them to nurture these relationships [88]. Increasing registered nurse staff hours may achieve better quality-indicator scores for pressure ulcers and use of physical restraints [89,90]. However, in the latter study, the ratio of nursing assistants to residents was not associated with rates of physical restraint use [90].

Under the federally mandated Long-Term Care Ombudsman Program (LTCOP), certified volunteer ombudsmen advocate for the welfare and rights of residents in NHs. These programs can be effective, but whether they are volunteer or paid may make a difference in effectiveness [91]. Findings from a nationwide study on factors associated with the perceived effectiveness of state LTCOPs showed that sufficient funding is positively associated with perceived effectiveness of work with NHs [92]. According to a descriptive study, volunteer ombudsmen felt most effective in promoting residents' rights and welfare and least effective in dealing with financial exploitation, nutrition, and hydration issues [93].

Although background checks take time and cost money, employers in NHs and home care may find them worthwhile. According to Susik [77], rough estimates from Florida suggest that up to 25% of all workers who apply for jobs in the home care industry have criminal records. This article implies that abuse of drugs by employees may lead to petty theft, absenteeism, financial exploitation, and physical abuse. Thus, "the best protection is an exhaustive screening, interviewing, and background checking process." Background checks can involve obtaining driving records, arrest records, or abuse records. Driving records can be obtained from the Department of Motor Vehicles through the mail with a signed release form and a small fee (about $3–$5). Procedures for inquiring about arrest records can be obtained by calling the local police department or sheriff's office and obtaining state law enforcement or criminal records. Records on individuals for whom a report of physical abuse or neglect has been confirmed are maintained by some states. Employers can contact state-funded social services departments to find out if their state has such databases. There are companies that specialize in doing background checks for job applicants, sometimes called "information brokers." They can be found in the Yellow Pages under titles such as "employment screening" or "employment consultants" or on the Internet under these titles and terms such as "background checks." Before doing background checks, it is critical to have the prospective employee sign a release form. There are four sample release forms in the article by Susik [77].

Education about aging can prevent ageism. Several methods can be used to debunk the myths of aging, including playing "The Aging Game"[94], reading books that give insight into how it is to live in a NH (eg, *Old Friends* [95]), or discussing well-known public personalities that continue to be successful into their 80s and 90s [96].

Education about elder abuse and neglect is necessary whether it is a discussion about definitions, risk factors, reporting, or how to prevent it [97]. All disciplines should have this area covered in their educational curriculum [98].

Home care workers are in a special position to evaluate and prevent elder abuse and neglect. However, they often face practical and ethical dilemmas, especially in cases of self-neglect, because older adults have a right to refuse services. It is in these cases where the multidisciplinary team approach is helpful on the patient's behalf and can help guide and give support to the home care worker dealing with the dilemma [18,99]. It is also in these circumstances where one author recommends "keeping a family focus" instead of a "rescuing focus" [71].

Summary

Elder abuse and neglect can be detected only through awareness, healthy suspicion, and knowledge of risk factors. A detailed and well-documented medical history, including information from the medical records, patient, family, and caregivers, and a comprehensive physical examination are necessary to identify and document signs of abuse and neglect. Suspected cases must be reported to adult protective services or other appropriate law enforcement agencies.

Elder abuse and neglect is a result of the dynamic interaction between personal, family, social and cultural values, priorities, and goals. Therefore, attention must be given to those factors that, although they do not cause abuse, contribute to its likelihood. In NHs, these risk factors include behavioral problems of the resident, staff caregiver burden, staff burnout, and staff ageism. In home care, risk factors include the personality problems of the family caregiver (more than overall caregiver burden), the characteristics of paid home care workers, and the psychosocial problems of the patient (eg, isolation, psychiatric illnesses, and poor social support). By its nature, abuse and neglect is person driven and preventable. Thus, patient and caregiver education and other interventions targeted toward risk factors or types of abuse or neglect play an invaluable role in preventing elder abuse and mistreatment.

References

[1] Fried LP, Ferrucci L, Darer J, et al. Untangling the concepts of disability, frailty, and comorbidity: implications for improved targeting and care. J Gerontol Med Sci 2004;59A: M255–63.

[2] Administration on Aging. Nursing Homes. Available at: www.aoa.gov/prof/notes/notes_nursing_homes.asp. Accessed July 17, 2004.

[3] Kane RL, Ouslander JG, Abrass IB. The essentials of clinical geriatrics. New York: McGraw-Hill; 2004.

[4] Leff B, Burton JR. The future history of home care and physician house calls in the United States. J Gerontol Med Sci 2001;56A:M603–8.

[5] Utech MR, Garret RR. Elder abuse and child abuse. Journal Interpersonal Violence 1992;7: 418–28.

[6] Fulmer TT, O'Malley TA. Inadequate care of the elderly. New York: Springer Publishing Company; 1987.

[7] Johnson T. Critical issues in the definition of elder mistreatment. In: Pillemer KA, Wolf S, editors. Elder abuse: conflict in the family. Dover, UK: Auburn House Publishing; 1986. p. 167–95.

[8] Hawes C, Kayser-Jones J. Abuse and neglect in nursing homes and institutions. Ann Long Term Care 2003;11:17–20.

[9] McDaniel CL. Elder abuse in institutional setting. Available at: www.keln.org/bibs/mcdaniel2.html. Accessed July 7, 2004.

[10] Hirst SP. Defining resident abuse within the culture of long-term care institutions. Clin Nurs Res 2002;11:267–84.

[11] Hirst SP. Resident abuse: an insider's perspective. Geriatr Nurs (Minneap) 2000;21:38–42.

[12] Spiegal C. Restraints, drugging rife in nursing homes. LA Times March 25, 1991:A1.

[13] Tousignant M, Davis P. Nursing homes in area, nationwide plagued by reports of abuse. Washington Post Oct. 13, 1996:B1.

[14] Eisler P. Dad's last days: tale of horror. USA Today Feb. 21, 1994:1A.

[15] Abuse of residents is a major problem in US nursing homes. Minority Staff Special Investigations Division, Committee on Government Reform, US House of Representatives, July 30, 2001. Available at: www.heaton.org/nursinghomesabuse.pdf. Accessed July 17, 2004.

[16] Pillemer K, Moore DW. Abuse of patients in nursing homes: findings from a survey of staff. Gerontologist 1989;29:314–20.

[17] Shugarman LR, Fries BE, Wolf RS, et al. Identifying older people at risk of abuse during routine screening practices. J Am Geriatr Soc 2003;51:24–31.

[18] Benton D, Marshall C. Elder buse. Clin Geriatr Med 1991;7:831–45.

[19] Burgess AW, Dowdell EB, Prentky RA. Sexual abuse of nursing home residents. J Psychosoc Nurs 2000;38:10–8.

[20] Marshall CE, Benton D, Brazier JM. Using clinical tools to identify clues of mistreatment. Geriatrics 2000;55:42–50.

[21] Payne BK, Cikovic R. An empirical examination of the characteristics, consequences, and causes of elder abuse in nursing homes. J Elder Abuse Negl 1995;7:61–74.

[22] Lachs MS, Williams C, O'Brien S, et al. Risk factors for reported elder abuse and neglect: a nine year observational cohort study. Gerontologist 1997;37:469–74.

[23] Grafstrom M, Nordberg A, Winblad B. Abuse is in the eye of the beholder: report by family members about abuse of demented persons in home care. A total population-based study. Scand J Soc Med 1993;21:247–55.

[24] Kosberg JI. Preventing elder abuse: identification of high risk factors prior to placement decisions. Gerontologist 1988;28:43–50.

[25] Goodridge DM, Johnson P, Thompson M. Conflict and aggression as stressors in the work environment of nursing assistants: implications for institutional elder abuse. J Elder Abuse Negl 1996;8:49–67.

[26] Meddough D. Convert elder abuse in nursing homes. J Elder Abuse Negl 1995;5:21–37.

[27] Jost BC, Grossberg GT. The evolution of psychiatric symptoms in Alzheimer's disease: a natural history study. J Am Geriatr Soc 1996;44:1078–81.

[28] Gubrium J. Living and dying at Murray Manor. New York: St. Martin's Press; 1975.

[29] Foner N. The caregiving dilemma: work in an American nursing home. Berkely (CA): University of California Press; 1994.

[30] Bowling A. Ageism in cardiology. BMJ 1999;319:1353–5.

[31] Mick DJ, Ackerman MH. Neutralizing ageism in critical care via outcomes research. AACN Clin Issues 1997;8:597–608.

[32] Grief CL. Patterns of ED use and perceptions of the elderly regarding their emergency care: a synthesis of recent research. J Emergency Nursing 2003;29:122–6.

[33] McCarthy P. Burnout in psychiatric nursing. J Adv Nurs 1985;10:305–10.

[34] Wierucka D, Goodridge D. Vulnerable in a safe place: institutional elder abuse. Can J Nurs Adm 1996;9:82–104.

[35] Matthias RE, Benjamin AE. Abuse and neglect of clients in agency-based and consumer-directed home care. Health Soc Work 2003;28:174–84.

[36] Krothe JS. Giving voice to elderly people: community-based long-term care. Public Health Nurs 1997;14:217–26.

[37] Macdonald NJ. Older nurses embrace hospice & home care. Caring 2004;23:50–1.

[38] Pillemer K, Bachman-Prehn R. Helping and hurting, predictors of maltreatment in nursing homes. Res Aging 1991;13:74–95.

[39] Pillemer K, Finkelhor D. Causes of elder abuse: caregiver stress versus problem relatives. Am J Orthopsychiatry 1989;59:179–87.

[40] Fulmer T, Guadagno L, Dyer CB, et al. Progress in elder abuse screening and assessment instruments. J Am Geriatr Soc 2004;52:297–304.

[41] Available at: www.oca.slu.edu/geriatricsyllabus/index.phtml?page=chapter1. Accessed July 22, 2004.

[42] Eisenberg DM, Davis RB, Ettner SL, et al. Trends in alternative medicine use in the United States, 1990–1997: results of a follow-up national survey. JAMA 1998;280:1569–75.

[43] Flaherty JH, Takahashi R, Teoh J, et al. Use of alternative therapies in older outpatients in the United States and Japan: prevalence, reporting patterns, and perceived effectiveness. J Gerontol Med Sci 2001;56:M650–5.

[44] Look KM, Look RM. Skin scraping, cupping, and moxibustion that may mimic physical abuse. J Forensic Sci 1997;42:103–5.

[45] Kane RS, Goodwin JS. Spontaneous fractures of the long bones in nursing home patients. Am J Med 1991;90:263–6.

[46] Chew DJ, Edmondson HD. A study of maxillofacial injuries in the elderly resulting from falls. J Oral Rehabil 1996;23:505–9.

[47] Akaza K, Bunai Y, Tsujinaka M, et al. Elder abuse and neglect: social problems revealed from 15 autopsy cases. Leg Med 2003;5:7–14.

[48] Burgess AW, Dowdell EB, Brown K. The elderly rape victim: stereotypes, perpetrators, and implications for practice. J Emerg Nurs 2000;26:516–8 [quiz 529].

[49] Morley JE, Kraenzle D. Causes of weight loss in a community nursing home. J Am Geriatr Soc 1994;42:583–5.

[50] Thomas DR, Ashmen W, Morley JE, et al. Nutritional management in long-term care: development of a clinical guideline. Council for Nutritional Strategies in Long-Term Care. J Gerontol Med Sci 2000;55:M725–34.

[51] Soini H, Routasalo P, Lagstrom H. Characteristics of the Mini-Nutritional Assessment in elderly home-care patients. Eur J Clin Nutr 2004;58:64–70.

[52] Davidhizar R, Dunn C. Malnutrition in the elderly. Home Healthcare Nurse 1996;14:948–54 [quiz 955–6].

[53] Suda Y, Marske CE, Flaherty JH, et al. Examining the effect of intervention to nutritional problems of the elderly living in an inner city area: a pilot project. J Nutr Health Aging 2001;5:118–23.

[54] Clark AN, Mankikar GD, Gray I. Diogenes syndrome: a clinical study of gross neglect in old age. Lancet 1975;1:366–8.

[55] Reyes-Ortiz CA. Diogenes syndrome: the self-neglect elderly. Compr Ther 2001;27:117–21.

[56] Cooney C, Hamid W. Review: Diogenes syndrome. Age Ageing 1995;24:451–3.

[57] Kiyak HA, Grayston MN, Crinean CL. Oral health problems and needs of nursing home residents. Community Dent Oral Epidemiol 1993;21:49–52.

[58] MacEntee MI. Oral care for successful aging in long-term care. J Public Health Dent 2000;60:326–9.

[59] McGee S, Abernethy WB, Simel DL. The rational clinical examination: is this patient hypovolemic? JAMA 1999;281:1022–9.

[60] Thomas DR, Tariq SH, Makhdomm S, et al. Physician misdiagnosis of dehydration in older adults. J Am Med Dir Assoc 2004;5:S30–4.

[61] Thomas DR. Are all pressure ulcers avoidable? J Am Med Dir Assoc 2003;4:S43–8.

[62] Pieper B, Templin TN, Dobal M, et al. Wound prevalence, types, and treatments in home care. Adv Wound Care 1999;12:117–26.

[63] Maklebust J. Preventing pressure ulcers in home care patients. Home Healthcare Nurse 1999;17:229–37 [quiz 237–8].

[64] Hiatt SW, Jones AA. Volunteer services for vulnerable families and at-risk elderly. Child Abuse Negl 2000;24:141–8.

[65] Clarke ME, Pierson W. Management of elder abuse in the emergency department. Emerg Med Clin North Am 1999;17:631–44.

[66] White SW. Elder abuse: critical care nurse role in detection. Crit Care Nurs Q 2000;23:20–5.

[67] Capezuti E, Brush BL, Lawson III WT. Reporting elder mistreatment. J Gerontol Nurs 1997; 23:24–32.

[68] Wolf RS, Li D. Factors affecting the rate of elder abuse reporting to a state protective services program. Gerontologist 1999;39:222–8.

[69] Lachs MS, Williams CS, O'Brien S, et al. Adult protective service use and nursing home placement. Gerontologist 2002;42:734–9.

[70] Hoban S, Kearney K. Elder abuse and neglect. It takes many forms: if you're not looking, you may miss it. Am J Nurs 2000;100:49–50.

[71] Hyde-Robertson B, Pirnie SM, Freeze C. A strategy against elderly mistreatment. Caring 1994;13:40–4.

[72] Agency on Aging. Elder abuse is a serious problem. Available at: www.aoa.gov/eldfam/Elder_ Rights/ Elder_Abuse/Elder_Abuse.asp. Accessed July 24, 2004.

[73] www.elderabusecenter.org/default.cfm?p=wheretoreportabuse.cfm. Accessed July 24, 2004.

[74] Amo MF, Rowe NL. Seven attributes of abuse prevention in long term care. Balance 2000; 4:6–10.

[75] Arvanis SC, Adelman RD, Breckman R, et al. Diagnostic and treatment guidelines on elder abuse and neglect. Arch Fam Med 1993;2:371–88.

[76] National Center on Elder Abuse. Available at: www.elderabusecenter.org/default.cfm. Accessed July 17, 2004.

[77] Susik DH. Background checks prevent abuse. Caring 1996;15:52–5.

[78] Beck C, Ortigara A, Mercer S, et al. Enabling and empowering certified nursing assistants for quality dementia care. Int J Geriatre Psychiatry 1999;14:197–211 [discussion 211–2].

[79] Peterson D, Berg-Weger MS, McGillick J, et al. Basic care I: the effect of dementia-specific training on certified nursing assistants and other staff. Am J Alzheimers Dis Other Demen 2002;17:154–64.

[80] Engelman KK, Altus DE, Mosier MC, et al. Brief training to promote the use of less intrusive prompts by nursing assistants in a dementia care unit. J Appl Behav Anal 2003;36:129–32.

[81] Gibson MC, MacLean J, Borrie M, et al. Orientation behaviors in residents relocated to a redesigned dementia care unit. Am J Alzheimers Dis Other Demen 2004;19:45–9.

[82] Cox H, Burns I, Savage S. Multisensory environments for leisure: promoting well-being in nursing home residents with dementia. J Gerontol Nurs 2004;30:37–45.

[83] van Weert JC, Kerkstra A, van Dulmen AM, et al. The implementation of snoezelen in psychogeriatric care: an evaluation through the eyes of caregivers. Int J Nurs Stud 2004;41: 397–409.

[84] Zeisel J, Silverstein NM, Hyde J, et al. Environmental correlates to behavioral health outcomes in Alzheimer's special care units. Gerontologist 2003;43:697–711.

[85] Werezak LJ, Morgan DG. Creating a therapeutic psychosocial environment in dementia care: a preliminary framework. J Gerontol Nurs 2003;29:18–25.

[86] The Greenhouse Project. Available at: www.thegreenhouseproject.com/index.htm. Accessed July 24, 2004.

[87] Annerstedt L. Group-living care: an alternative for the demented elderly. Demen Geriatr Cogn Disord 1997;8:136–42.

[88] Bowers BJ, Esmond S, Jacobson N. The relationship between staffing and quality in long-term care facilities: exploring the views of nurse aides. J Nurs Care Qual 2000;14:55–64 [quiz 73–5].

[89] Bostick JE. Relationship of nursing personnel and nursing home care quality. J Nurs Care Qual 2004;19:130–6.

[90] Castle NG. Nursing homes with persistent deficiency citations for physical restraint us. Med Care 2002;40:868–78.

[91] Netting FE, Huber R, Kautz III JR. Volunteer and paid long term care ombudsmen: differences in complaint resolution. J Volunt Adm 1995;13:10–21.

[92] Estes CL, Zulman DM, Goldberg SC, et al. State long term care ombudsman programs: factors associated with perceived effectiveness. Gerontologist 2004;44:104–15.

[93] Ostwald SK, Runge A, Lees EJ, et al. Texas certified volunteer Long-Term Care Ombudsmen: perspectives of role and effectiveness. J Am Med Dir Assoc 2003;4:323–8.

[94] McVey LJ, Davis DE, Cohen HJ. The 'aging game': an approach to education in geriatrics. JAMA 1989;262:1507–9.

[95] Kidder T. Old friends. Boston: Houghton Mifflin; 1993.

[96] Available at: www.oca.slu.edu/geriatricsyllabus/index.phtml?page=chapter2. Accessed July 25, 2004.

[97] Scogin F, Stephens G, Bynum J. Training caregivers: the development of an elder abuse prevention program. J Health Hum Resource Adm 1990;12:499–508.

[98] Laditka SB, Fischer M, Mathews KB, et al. There's no place like home: evaluating family medicine residents' training in home care. Home Health Care Serv Q 2002;21:1–17.

[99] Wolf RS, Pillemer K. What's new in elder abuse programming? Four bright ideas. Gerontologist 1994;34:126–9.

ELSEVIER
SAUNDERS

Clin Geriatr Med 21 (2005) 355–364

CLINICS IN
GERIATRIC
MEDICINE

Cultural Issues and Elder Mistreatment

Anne R. Simpson, MD, CMD*

Division of Geriatrics, Department of Internal Medicine,
The University of New Mexico Health Sciences Center, School of Medicine,
MSC11 6095, Albuquerque, NM 87131, USA

We are at the dawn of a new social construct that is unlike any other that we have known. Our population is aging at a rapid pace, and we continue to battle the deleterious effects of poverty, substance dependence, and a multitude of other societal ills. Many of these changes have resulted in significant alterations in family and socio-cultural dynamics. Our elders are faced with longer years and a blurred vision of what those years hold in store for them. We have a large number of elders who are the primary caregivers for their young (adolescent and younger) family members. In addition to providing for others, they are dealing with their own chronic illnesses and a lack of adequate financial support. At the opposite end of this picture is the elder who has lost her younger generation of family members to violence, substance dependence, and so forth, and now has joined the category of the "unbefriended elder." Another increasingly familiar scenario is that of the frail elder acting as primary caregiver for their frail aged loved one. These situations and numerous others reflect a population of people who are vulnerable and at significant risk for elder mistreatment. To prevent the occurrence of elder mistreatment, one needs to define it and to identify causal and cultural relationships that may play a role in it and to educate entire communities about it.

Elder mistreatment is defined as abuse, neglect, exploitation, and violation of rights. Abuse can be physical, emotional, or psychologic. Box 1 lists definitions of the various forms of elder abuse.

---

* Institute for Ethics, MSC11 6095, Albuquerque, NM 87131-0001.
E-mail address: asimpson@salud.unm.edu

0749-0690/05/$ – see front matter © 2005 Elsevier Inc. All rights reserved.
doi:10.1016/j.cger.2004.11.003   *geriatric.theclinics.com*

Box 1. Forms of elder abuse

- Physical abuse: An act of violence in which the perpetrator intentionally inflicts pain or injury on the elder
- Emotional or psychologic abuse: Intentionally berating, threatening, isolating, or causing emotional harm to the elder
- Neglect: The act of withholding resources (physical, psychologic, or financial) that the elder needs for health and well-being
- Exploitation: Use of the elder's material resources for the personal gain of others
- Violation of rights: The act of over-riding the wishes and desires of the elder when the elder has the decisional capability for self-determination

---

The above list forms a basic definition of elder mistreatment that is recognized by the medical community. Elder mistreatment also is recognized as a criminal offense, and each state carries its own definition of elder mistreatment in the criminal context. Some states, such as New Mexico, have made the failure to report elder mistreatment a criminal offense [1].

Although a lot of attention has been directed toward dealing with issues of elder mistreatment, its incidence continues to grow. This can be reflective of the rising number of people who are living longer and growing older, but it can also be reflective of the level of ignorance that surrounds this subject. There are times when members of a health care team fail to recognize or acknowledge situations of elder mistreatment. This is particularly true when the situation is occurring among members of a nondominant culture group. This does not seem to represent condoning the behavior but instead shows a discomfort with cultural competence in issues of elder mistreatment. Several scholarly publications have printed reports of research on elder mistreatment in minority populations. The prevailing themes that flow through the literature and that are identified as risk factors for mistreatment in these communities include poverty and its consequences, isolation, lack of access to health care, stress, and dependency. Griffin's study on elder abuse in the African American population [2] and Carson and Hand's study of elder abuse in the Native American population [3] refer to the history of trauma and abuse that has been inflicted on these populations. In these populations, physical and psychologic abuse was used to punish and exploit, which is a factor that has contributed to mistreatment in these populations. It is easy to blame the dominant culture as a major contributor to the mistreatments that occur in these communities, but the picture is complex and requires an assessment of a multitude of factors that are beyond the scope of this article. There is, however, a significant element that requires consideration when one is addressing the issue of elder mistreatment, and that is culture. What role does culture play in elder mistreatment? Our deeply imbedded interpretation of the world and how we function in it is due in part to our cultural beliefs and value system. These things were learned from our parents and grandparents and shape many of our actions and interactions and give us a sense of who we are.

Mrs. Z was a 93-year-old woman whom I treated in my medical practice. She was a widow with five children and many grandchildren and great grandchildren. She described herself as a "traditional Mexican American," and her lifestyle seemed to reflect those values. As she progressed in age, Mrs. Z developed dementia in addition to her other chronic illnesses. She required around-the-clock care. She was receiving excellent care from her daughters: Her eldest daughter lived with her and served as the primary caregiver, and the other daughters provided respite care. I made routine home visits. Things seemed to be going well until Mrs. Z developed pneumonia and needed hospitalization. She recovered fairly quickly from the illness but was weak and deconditioned and needed rehabilitation therapy to regain her level of functioning. It was at this point that the question of where she should get her therapy became a major issue for her children. Her sons felt that Mrs. Z should return home and receive home-based therapy, whereas her daughters had a different view of the plan. Mrs. Z's eldest daughter, who was also an elder, had been living with and providing care for Mrs. Z. This daughter reported that she was under treatment for several chronic conditions herself, and although her sisters were supportive and provided respite care for their mother, it was not enough. The eldest daughter was a widow and did not have children of her own, so the family saw her as the natural caregiver for Mrs. Z. The other two daughters had husbands, children, and grandchildren to manage and therefore were not available to provide anything more than respite care for their mother. Mrs. Z's two sons, according to their sisters, were not directly involved in the care of their mother, but out of tradition they were the decision makers for her. Based on traditional values, their decision was to have their mother return home in the care of the older sister.

As a physician and advocate for my patient, my role took on a complexity of ethical, moral, and legal considerations. It was clear to me that discharging Mrs. Z to her home environment would jeopardize her health and well-being and that of her eldest daughter. As I weighed the basic principles of ethics, the navigation of the situation became less daunting. Mrs. Z's son's had the legal authority, in the form of a Power of Attorney, to have her care provided in the home environment, but this was not in the best interest of the patient. The eldest daughter had admitted that she was unable to provide the care that was needed, so if I sent her home, I would knowingly be sending her into a potentially unsafe environment. The first goal was to do no harm to either party. The sons were opposed to having their mother placed in a long-term care facility because it had not been part of their cultural practice. I explained to the sons that it was my opinion that their mother would not get the level of care that she needed at home; she needed rehab at a long-term care facility. I recommended a facility that had an excellent reputation. The family went out to visit the facility and agreed to the placement. This seemed to be right thing to do under the circumstances. During one of my follow-up conversations with Mrs. Z's daughters, they explained that my intervention and medical opinion had influenced their brothers and their cultural community.

In this case, there seemed to be two potential victims: Mrs. Z and her eldest daughter. Mrs. Z was at risk for physical and psychologic abuse associated with caregiver stress, and she was also at risk for neglect. On the other hand, her daughter was a setup for exploitation, neglect by others, and self-neglect. It is likely that these forms of abuse were already occurring. It seemed clear to me that the family was not aware of any of these issues. They were following a long-treaded cultural path in an attempt to provide care for there aged and disabled mother. In doing so, they were teetering on the edge of committing one or more criminal acts because their cultural practice did not support the letter of the law. A recent report by Stanford [4] addressed this issue as follows:

> ... The mixing of values, traditions and various cultural practices has made it necessary to consciously try to understand and contemplate how to maximize the social, economic and political benefits of bringing together multiple cultures. Any operating body must understand that as cultures merge and undergo change there is a constant sloughing off of artifacts that distinguish cultures. However, there is also a tenaciousness about holding on to those things that distinguish culture. The artifacts and social behaviors that distinguish cultures within different environments are those elements that cause us to recognize diversity. ...

Historically, our population has been in flux with immigrants from around the world establishing residencies here on a daily basis, and this has led to a truly diverse society. As families establish themselves, they face a significant amount of stress looking for employment, finding affordable housing and transportation, dealing with language barriers, and so forth. This can be daunting for elders who may now be isolated and totally dependent on their children and grand-children for financial and social support. In some of these families, the children find jobs and the grandchildren go off to school, leaving the elder alone, isolated, and responsible for household chores. The family's culture may see this as communal support, but others may see it as social isolation and exploitation of labor; this is especially true if the elder is sad and desires to return home.

The literature on elder mistreatment in minority populations recognizes exploitation as a form of abuse; however, in some situations there is a caveat to consider. Griffin [2] points out that there is "... a type of symbiotic or mutually beneficial relationship that can be found in African American communities. The elders seem to have an understanding, an unwritten contract, with their adult child or grandchild to provide financial support, housing, etc. in return for the younger persons continued presence in the home."

As African Americans in rural Alabama, my family and the community held those same expectations. When I was growing up, segregation and the job situation forced adult children to look elsewhere for employment; however the expectation was that the children would return home to care for the aged parents when it was necessary. I questioned my mother about this practice, noting that the adult child would not be able to make a financial contribution if they returned home to this rural environment. My mother's response surprised me. She said, "If the parent can live on that small sum so can the child, and the child should be happy to do so." The community in which we lived was composed of several people who were one generation removed from slavery, and their belief system was based, in part, on religious faith. People believed that God would make a way in every situation. Therefore, sharing meager amounts with one's kin was not seen as exploitation—it was a way to maintain life and a level of freedom. There were clearly situations in which the elder was exploited, their funds were taken, and care was not provided. This was seen as a violation of an unwritten cultural law, but the punishment was expected to come from God and nowhere else. The adult child's return to the home for the sole purpose of caring for the elder is honorable, but it is exploitative of the child and can be stressful. It is also a risk factor for elder mistreatment. Community and family expectations can be a tremendous burden to bear. Armed with an appreciation for cultural diversity and the associated expectations, I address these issues in my practice as a method of abuse prevention. Working with patients and their families together, we can explore options that may be considered as reasonable in their cultural framework. This can be a trying task but well worth the effort if it prevents an act of mistreatment.

Having family members return home is not a practice that is particular to one cultural community. Brown [5] documents this practice in the Navajo community. He states in his article that "Income was a 'catch-22' phenomenon for the elderly Navajos.... it was a matter of their voluntarily sharing what they had with family members who had needs. To them it was clearly a case of living up to an important cultural value."

The identification of financial exploitation as a form of abuse can be complicated at best; however, there are a number of states in which the health care providers are expected to recognize and report all forms of elder mistreatment. In those states, exploitation is listed as a form of mistreatment, but health care providers have not been trained to identify the problem. The elders and their families are finding themselves caught between the law and their cultural beliefs. Some of the considerations that face elders in poverty can be seen as a matter of life or death: Should money be used to pay for medication for the elder, or should it be used to support the education of a grandchild? In poverty-stricken communities, this is an important question and can leave one between self-neglect and hope for the future.

> Diverse groups, issues, environments and cultural practices shape our society. The United States was purportedly founded on the basis of inclusion. The founding fathers did not correctly envision the changes in gender, color, general environment and levels of functioning of individuals in society. The Constitution and other historical documents were based on a smaller male Euro-descendent population. There was no thought given to including American Indians, Americans of African descent, Asian-Americans or Hispanics. Each major group cited has moved into the mainstream and is very much a part of the decision-making process for determining what is considered to be an appropriate lifestyle in America [4].

Elder abuse is a recognized offense regardless of the ethnicity of the victim and the perpetrator; this was made clear when researchers interviewed older persons from different cultural groups, comparing attitudes about elder mistreatment. The researchers found that there were differences in how different cultural groups defined abuse. Two examples of the types of questions and the response are as follows: "[Responding to 37 possible abuse scenarios,] [t]he Native Americans ranked [four] more items as abusive and 22 items at a higher level of severity than did the African Americans, who rated [three] more items as abusive and 15 as more severe than did the Caucasians" [6]. "Korean American elderly respondents held significantly more negative attitudes toward involvement of persons outside the family in elder abuse incidents, as well as toward reporting of such incidents to the authorities and the consequences for perpetrators" [6].

Although elder mistreatment is identified somewhat differently across cultures, it is a situation to be reckoned with on at least two levels: the root causes and the failure to report. There has been a noticeable concern in the literature regarding under-reporting of elder mistreatment. This is an issue that seems to be prevalent across cultures, and there have been a number of reasons listed for this phenomenon. Among the list of reasons are low self-esteem, shame, fear of retaliation, dependency, fear of placement in a long-term care facility, and fear of reprisal from the perpetrator.

People are ashamed and embarrassed to find themselves victims of abuse. Victims are often seen as weak and powerless in our society. Elders during "usual aging" generally experience a decline in there sensory and motor strength and their vitality. No matter how expected these conditions are, no one seems to be prepared to accept the body and mind changes that accompany aging. The victim may be reluctant to report abuses and to discuss their age-associated disabilities for fear that they will be placed in a long-term care facility. Elders, like other members of society, want to be seen as strong and capable when it applies to providing self-care. It can be especially difficult to report a perpetrator who is a trusted friend or family member.

There is also the situation where the victim has been the perpetrator of abuse and is now the victim; this is part of what is described as the "cycle of violence." The cycle of violence for many cultures, including Native American and African American, has an associated history that is rife with acts of violence perpetrated by the dominant culture.

> ...The mind set of many social scientists and others is that what has happened to many minority older people is in the distant past. The laws and policies that were established to control the lifestyles and activities of individuals of nearly a century ago have a continuing effect on older people of today. The history that we often speak of is not a distant history; it is a very recent history. Abuse is said to exist across generations in families, and families make up communities and society. If this type of analogy is accurate, it becomes clear that macro abuse that has had an impact on older people who were born close to the turn of the century will continue to have some impact on three or more generations hence" [4].

This statement leads me to further reflect on my childhood days in Alabama where children who misbehaved were subjected to physical abuse at the hands of their parents. In some African American communities, corporal punishment was considered an essential component of child rearing. The prevailing thought was that it was a parent's duty to introduce the child to what may befall them should their behavior continue and, most especially, if their "bad behavior" offended members of the "white" society. This was looked upon as a lesson because it was felt that a parent, in their act of corporal punishment, would not be as harsh as the "white man" and therefore would not cause harm or death to the child. This is just one of the lessons learned from slavery that continues to haunt us through the cycle of violence.

An a priori reason for why some people do not report episodes of mistreatment is the ongoing history of how minorities are treated by the criminal justice system. In spite of the fact that an elder is being mistreated, they may still love and want to protect the perpetrator from the abuse of the criminal justice system. There is also the fear of agencies. "Members of WE ARE FAMILY noted that family members have a tendency to 'pull out' or abandon elderly relatives when agencies get involved" [7].

This type of fear can explain why neighbors are afraid to report cases of mistreatment. People do not want to get involved because they do not know the circumstances of the family. This can be especially true if the neighborhood is known to house undocumented workers. Undocumented elders are a particularly vulnerable segment of the population; they have a significantly high set of risk factors. They tend to be isolated, lack assess to health care, have low self-esteem (often because of language barriers), are often dependent on others, and are not likely to report the perpetrator for fear of deportation. They often live under poverty conditions. There is a plurality of reasons for not reporting elder abuse, just as there is a plurality of victims and perpetrators.

The discussion thus far has focused on a few ethnic cultures, and the few that have been mentioned need to be further examined to consider the subcultures housed in each group. There is not a singular Native American culture; there are hundreds of Native tribal and pueblo communities, each with its own cultural values. This concept applies to other ethnic group; there are a multitude of subheadings under the rubric for each ethnic group. This needs to be considered whenever one looks at issues of culture, ethnicity, and diversity. It would be inappropriate to presume the ethnicity and culture of an individual based solely on their physical appearance. If cultural information is needed, it is appropriate to ask.

There are a host of cultures that are rarely mentioned in the literature on elder mistreatment but that are viable growing populations with aging generations among them. Some of those groups are the disabled community, the deaf community, the gay/lesbian/transgender community, the community of undocumented workers, and many religious communities.

Elder mistreatment has been recognized in these communities at micro and macro levels. Micro refers to conditions that affect a small number of peo-

ple and are more personal in nature. Macro refers to conditions that have
an impact on a wide range of people and can be put in place through legislation or policy [4]. These populations are prime targets for elder mistreatment at multiple levels. They tend to be isolated or ostracized from
mainstream society.

An example of a macro element of elder mistreatment including social
negligence and isolation where the dominant culture is the perpetrator occurs
in the deaf community. The deaf community's isolation is related to a language
barrier. The members of the community cannot hear spoken language, and their
communication skills take on different forms. Members of the hearing
community have done little to recognize the culture of the deaf community. In
our failure to acknowledge another community culture, we place ourselves at
increasingly greater distances from that population; in so doing, we deny access
to care to members of the other community.

We also deny access to assessment of and education on the topic of elder
mistreatment and other subjects. Many health care environments are sensitive
to language differences and recruit employees who speak languages that are
common to the community. However, to my knowledge, sign language and deaf
culture competency are not widely recognized by the dominant culture. There
may be acts of elder mistreatment occurring within the deaf community, but I am
not aware of research that has been done on that subject.

The next group that has to be addressed is the lesbian, gay male, and trans-
gender community. Members of this community have been battered, maimed, and
killed for no other reason than the fact that they exist. This in itself isolates
the gay elder from the dominant community. Fearing the outcomes, individuals
are afraid to disclose their sexual orientation to members of the dominant culture. This can be especially true for elders who may have lived a lifetime hiding
a part of their life that held personal meaning and value at the deepest level.
These elders are at risk for exploitation through blackmail and other means.
They can be threatened with the idea of having the life they have protected
revealed to others. Some may find themselves estranged from their birth families
and at risk of becoming "unbefriended" should they lose their partner or social
support system.

There have been a few reports on domestic violence in same-sex relationships.
When people age, their patterned behavior may not change, and the violence
that occurred at a younger age is likely to continue in the later years. There are
also reports that have shown victims becoming aggressive as the perpetrator's
health status declines. Domestic violence is alive in the geriatric population and
it has no cultural boundaries.

There are people who, by choice or circumstances, find themselves alone
during the later years of life. People who fit this category are from diverse
cultural and ethnic backgrounds, but what they have in common is an absence
of friends and family; they are the "unbefriended" elders. In my practice as a
geriatrician, I have been introduced to members of this population most often
through the Adult Protective Service Agency. These elders have been reported

through various sources because of exploitation, battery, self-neglect, and so forth. A number of the people whom I have taken care of under these circumstances have been diagnosed with a dementia and have required protective custody because they lacked decisional capacity. Placing an elder in a sheltered environment protects the individual and the community. The sheltered environment should have as few restrictions as possible to permit the maximal amount of freedom with minimal risks for the elder.

Elder mistreatment in most states is a criminal offense, and laws have been designed to protect the victim and prosecute the perpetrator. The legal system has demonstrated its abhorrence of these crimes by implementing mandatory reporting laws in some states. The passing of legislative acts sends a clear message that elder mistreatment is not tolerated by the legal system. The message that is going out is a legal one, but the issues have multiple components, including that of public health. Elder mistreatment is a disease process that afflicts many systems, and it has an increasing morbidity and mortality rate. This particular social illness needs to be addressed with methods that are implemented whenever there is menacing disease process active in the environment.

> Public health accountability addresses the responsibility of public health agents to work with the public and scientific experts to identify, define, and understand at a fundamental level the threats to public health, and the risks and benefits of ways to address them. The appropriate level of public involvement in the analytic-deliberative process depends on the particular public health problem [8].

For well over a decade, some Native American communities have been actively engaged in passing tribal laws to protect their elders. They are also promoting culturally sensitive community education on the issues of elder mistreatment. The Navajo Tribe have produced a Navajo language video that is use to educate the elders and other members of the community. The indigenous filmmaker Phil Lucas and the Oregon Department of Human Services have produced a video entitled "Restoring the Sacred Circle, Responding to Elder Abuse in American Indian Communities" [9]. There have been community forums on the topic and the distribution of written materials that are reflective of a multimedia campaign to inform the community and to protect the elders who are with us and future generations of elders [10].

The work that is being done in some Native American communities is exemplary and demonstrates an approach that can be taken to facilitate a community recovery. The treatment involved a community education project that was culture and language specific; multiple forms of conveyance were used. The people who delivered the messages were members of the cultural community for whom the message was intended. A similar type of project can be developed and implemented in other communities to address elder mistreatment as a public health concern. Public awareness is the first step toward recovery from this disease. Elders in our country are subject to these risks; we all will be, in our later years, if the status quo remains.

References

[1] New Mexico Resident Abuse and Neglect Act of 1978 [30-47-1 to 30-47-10 NMSA].
[2] Griffin LW. Elder maltreatment in the African American community: you just don't hit your momma!!! In: Tatara T, editor. Understanding elder abuse in minority populations. Philadelphia: Taylor & Francis; 1998. p. 27–45.
[3] Carson DK, Hand C. Dilemmas surrounding elder abuse and neglect in Native American communities. In: Tatara T, editor. Understanding elder abuse in minority populations. Philadelphia: Taylor & Francis; 1998. p. 161–80.
[4] Stanford EP. Diversity in an aging society: abuse the wild card. In: Understanding and combating elder abuse in minority communities. Long Beach (CA): Archstone Foundation; 1998. p. 19–24.
[5] Brown AS. Patterns of abuse among Native American elderly. In: Tatara T, editor. Understanding elder abuse in minority populations. Philadelphia: Taylor & Francis; 1998. p. 143–58.
[6] Hudson MF, Carlson JR. Elder abuse: its meaning to Caucasians, African Americans and Native Americans. In: Tatara T, editor. Understanding elder abuse in minority populations. Philadelphia: Taylor & Francis; 1998. p. 187–203.
[7] Nerenberg L. Culturally specific outreach. In: Understanding and combating elder abuse in minority communities. Long Beach (CA): Archstone Foundation; 1998. p. 152–67.
[8] Childress JF, Faden RR, Gaare RD, et al. Public health ethics: mapping the terrain. J Law Med Ethics 2002;30:170–8.
[9] Phil Lucas Productions. Restoring the sacred circle: responding to elder abuse in American Indian communities [video]. Issaquah (WA): Oregon Department of Human Services; 2002.
[10] Honor the keeper of the beauty: an injury prevention project. Gallup (NM): Gallup Indian Medical Center.

Further readings

Jogerst GJ, Daly JM, Brinig MF, et al. Domestic elder abuse and the law. Am J Public Health 2003; 93:2131–6.

Kapp MB. Criminal and civil liability of physicians for institutional elder abuse and neglect. J Am Med Dir Assoc 2002;2(Suppl):576–81.

Maguire P. Why the nation's toughest elder abuse laws make some California physicians nervous. American College of Physicians. ACP-ASIM Observer, March 2003. Available at: www.acponline.org. Accessed January 21, 2005.

Themes from a grounded theory analysis of elder neglect assessment by experts. Gerontologist 2002;43:745–52.

ELSEVIER
SAUNDERS

Clin Geriatr Med 21 (2005) 365–382

CLINICS IN
GERIATRIC
MEDICINE

When Elders Lose their Cents: Financial Abuse of the Elderly

Kimberly Reed, RN, JD, LLM

*Elder Law and Estate Planning, Reed Law Associates, P.C., 555 Skokie Boulevard, Suite 500,
Northbrook, IL 60062, USA*

Case 1

Mr. S. was a spry 92-year-old widower who loved nothing more than a good evening of dancing and camaraderie at the local community center. More often than not, a woman in her fifties was also in attendance at these get-togethers in town, and she would indulge Mr. S's penchant for a good dance around the floor. Dancing and dinner turned into weekend trips and became week-long trips to places in the United States and then to Europe. His family wondered out loud about the intentions of this woman, but Mr. S. had always been a private man, and they were satisfied that he had things under control. "After all, they aren't getting married or anything," the family would say. When Mr. S. died suddenly, the family was shocked to find this woman had transferred all of Mr. S.'s bank accounts to her individual name with a Power of Attorney apparently signed by Mr. S. shortly into their relationship. By the time the family discovered the problem, the woman was long gone with all of Mr. S.'s hard-earned assets.

Case 2

Mrs. H.'s 52-year-old son had never held a job longer than 6 months in his adult life. He lived most of his life with his parents in the large family home. When Mr. H. died, leaving a several million dollar estate, the son assured his siblings he would take care of their mother, reminding them "you both have

E-mail address: Reedlaw408@aol.com

families and I don't." When Mrs. H.'s Alzheimer disease progressed to early-mid stage, she was admitted to an assisted living facility on the recommendation of her physician and with the siblings' concurrence but over the vehement protests of the at-home son. Three weeks after moving into the facility, Mrs. H. announced to her other children that her son would be buying a "bigger and better home" for the two of them to live in because "Bobby says this place is just not right." At that point, the oldest son began checking and found his brother had systematically transferred assets from his mother's bank accounts, sold her investments, and had made a down payment on a multi-million dollar condominium unit in the heart of the large nearby city, nowhere near where Mrs. H. had lived before.

Case 3

Jane was the married secretary to the wealthy Mr. P. who was 44 years her senior. She began an affair with him, eventually divorcing her husband and marrying the widowed Mr. P. The adult children from his first marriage were immediately prevented from contacting Mr. P. through Jane's manipulations and nonstop efforts of estrangement, at one point lying to Mr. P. that his adult children were so mad at him for marrying her they did not want to see him ever again. Jane deliberately organized Mr. P's days in and out of the office. When a stroke and hip replacement forced his complete retirement, Jane stepped up control over her husband, reducing his activities to a carefully chosen two or three activities per day, all within the confines of the grounds of their large, often-remodeled, and expanded house. Meanwhile, the adult children tried desperately to contact their father, enlisting the help of their father's oldest and dearest friends who were finally able to get in and break the cycle of control. By that time, Jane had reduced Mr. P.'s multi-million holdings to a relative pittance while her own separate accounts had swelled proportionately.

These cases illustrate only a few of the many ways elder financial abuse can happen. As aging baby boomers become the majority of the population, elder abuse in all of its forms will be more prevalent. Recognizing the overt and the subtle signs of abuse is important for all professionals dealing with the elderly.

Of the major categories of abuse identified by the National Center on Elder Abuse (NCEA) [1], financial abuse is one of the hardest forms of abuse to recognize. With physical abuse, there are bruises or weight loss, and there are behavioral changes with emotional or psychologic abuse. The signs of financial abuse may not register with anyone, least of all the elder, until it is well advanced. As with the other types of abuse, the abuser may be anyone—a family member, a caregiver/care taker, or a complete stranger who finagles his/her way into the vulnerable senior's life. Therein lies the problem: There is no consistently "typical" victim, and there is no consistently "typical" perpetrator.

Because elder financial mistreatment or abuse can happen anywhere there is an elder, prevalence of abusive actions is hard to quantify; many studies have made an attempt, and it is an ongoing endeavor [2–4]. Without a universally agreed-upon definition of "elder financial abuse," the sheer size of the potential study population, and differences in research methodology, studies analyze data describing different aspects without analyzing the problem as a whole, resulting in inaccuracies or under-reporting. In addition to research inconsistencies, there are problems with obtaining the raw data. The victimized elder may feel embarrassed as a result of the loss or intimidated by the abuser, or the reporter of the alleged abuse (the victim or third party) may be worried about retribution of an abuse report. Health care professionals may not be aware there is an abuse issue if the victim cannot or will not make a report or if the professional is not attuned to the symptoms of abuse.

Definition

Elder financial abuse is also known as "financial mistreatment" and "financial exploitation." There are many shades of this problem. Financial abuse can be an "improper act or process of an individual, using the resources of an older person without his/her consent, for someone else's benefit" [5] or unintended account misuse or withholding of resources by a third party. Financial abuse can be the concealment of belongings or money. Also included under the heading of financial abuse are fraud, embezzlement, undue influence, and misuse of guardianship/conservatorship and Powers of Attorney [6].

The fact the elder victim may not be able to see or hear well makes them an easy target. If a caregiver, family member, or a "kind" stranger is asked by the elder to help sign a check or fill out a form containing financial information, the temptation to engage in financial abuse may be irresistible to one so inclined. These same people may offer their "help" to the elder, thereby gaining the necessary information to access financial accounts. If the elder is unable to oversee the correctness of the transaction, he may not realize his helper has just removed funds right out from under him. Also, the relative liquidity of assets (eg, stocks, bonds, insurance policies, and property) makes access or transfer with a coerced Power of Attorney, with a forged signature, or through undue influence fairly easy. The abuser can be almost anyone in the elder's life. Although the abuser is usually a family member or a significant other, anyone in a position of authority or trust should be suspected when financial abuse is an issue [7]. These people might include the elder's caregiver or a professional, such as a lawyer, doctor, accountant, banker, or a stranger who is "kind and caring" [7].

Identification

Often, financial abuse goes undetected for a long period of time. It may start off on a small scale, perhaps one or two episodes over a period of a few months, and then escalate as the elder becomes more trusting or the episodes go

---

Box 1. Evidence of financial abuse

- Accumulation of unpaid bills
- Unusual or sudden changes in banking activity
- Loss of valuable possessions without explanation
- Sudden changes made to estate planning documents (eg, addition or removal of beneficiary names)
- The elder's own statements about lack of funds or suspicions of theft

---

unnoticed. The abuser may isolate the elder to the point where the elder is in the complete control of the abuser. Box 1 lists forms of evidence of financial abuse.

Outward signs of elder financial abuse may include the receipt of unnecessary services, goods, or subscriptions. Classic home-improvement scams ("My crew is in the neighborhood, and we're inspecting and repairing roofs before the winter comes. We've got a special going right now to do this work for you, but we can only offer this special price today...") are an example of financial abuse by strangers. There may be a sudden close personal relationship with a much younger or able person that may involve marriage or cohabitation. Medical conditions such as malnutrition, dehydration, or declining health in general may be indirect signs of financial abuse if the elder does not have sufficient funds to purchase food or medicine. Changes in lifestyle (becoming reclusive, appearing to make unusual types or numbers of purchases) or lack of amenities (no television, inappropriate clothing for the season) should trigger suspicions of financial abuse if there is no other obvious explanation.

Consumer fraud affects everyone, including the elderly. The scams foisted on seniors include health and life insurance fraud, telemarketing fraud, securities fraud, mail order fraud, and home improvement-related or home loan/equity scams. Elders are often easy prey because of diminished hearing or mental capacity and may be easily influenced. Consumer fraud against the elderly population is not often reported due to embarrassment and uncertainty of where and how to report the scam. The fact that an entire life's savings can be lost to one enterprising con artist makes consumer fraud a particularly heinous crime.

The most common evidence of financial abuse involves unusual banking activity, forged signatures, depletion of savings, and interception of income checks [4]. Misuse of Powers of Attorney documents are one way the abuser gains access to an elder's financial information and accounts. In other cases, the elder simply complies with the abuser's demands for funds. Financial institutions are usually not liable for honoring what seems to be a valid Power of Attorney document. In Illinois, for example, see 755 ILCS 45/2–8: "Any person who acts in good faith reliance on a copy of the agency will be fully protected and released to the same extent as though the reliant had dealt directly with the named principal as a fully-competent person." Increased credit card usage may be another sign of abuse.

As with most forms of elder abuse, financial abuse or exploitation has at its root a trusting or confidential relationship between the elder and the abuser. When this fiduciary relationship exists, a careful look should be given to any unusual financial activity, such as a large gift or transfer of ownership of a major asset to someone who may not normally be an expected donee of such an item.

Legal aspects

Financial abuse usually leaves a paper trail. Review of bank statements, credit card statements, ATM receipts, or usage records can paint a clear picture of financial abuse. Any increase in the number of withdrawals by an elder who is home bound or unable to write is a tip-off to abuse. Likewise, review of legal documents, such as Powers of Attorney for Property or deeds and tax returns, might reveal a history of abuse when the elder is unwilling or unable to assist in an investigation.

Once discovered, financial abuse can be remedied with various legal actions including conversion, recision, accounting, and voidance. Conversion is the unauthorized assumption of ownership of property. Rescission is the annulment or cancellation of a contract. An accounting in a financial abuse setting would include the court-ordered determination of a balance due and usually includes the requirement to pay the amount due. Voidance is the determination that a contract or agreement is null or having no legal force. These legal actions may recover the actual asset, the value of the asset, or restore the elder to the way he was before the abuse. Other civil actions may include breach of fiduciary duty, negligence, undue influence, and intentional infliction of emotional distress.

Of these actions, undue influence is perhaps one of the hardest to describe and prove. In the simplest sense, it is any situation in which the elder is prevented from exercising his own free will and judgment The legal definition is "persuasion, pressure or influence short of actual force, but stronger than mere advice, that so overpowers the dominated party's free will or judgement that he or she cannot act intelligently and voluntarily, but act instead, subject to the will or purposes of the dominating party" [8]. Proving undue influence has occurred is difficult because the burden of proof is on the elder, the one who alleges it took place. If the elder cannot or does not cooperate in describing how he was unduly or improperly influenced and by whom, it is difficult to bring a lawsuit.

Criminal causes of action may also be appropriate in cases of financial abuse. There are a wide range of criminal statutes in place throughout the country.

Financial exploitation may be prosecuted as actions for theft, burglary, forgery, mail fraud, possession of stolen property, extortion, and embezzlement. Even with a fair number of causes of action available, there are few prosecutions for criminal financial abuse because of under-reporting resulting from the fact that abusers tend to be family members or from the victim being unable or unwilling to describe the criminal activities [10–14].

An extra set of eyes to help detect and prosecute this type of abuse would be helpful. Professionals in the banking community, for example, can be on the lookout for activity indicative of financial exploitation of elderly account holders. In addition, fiduciary abuse specialty teams composed of accountants, FBI agents, insurance claims detectives, and other specialists can root out instances of financial exploitation before the situation gets out of hand [9].

Criminal penalties for abuse are on the books in about half of the states and are usually found within state adult protective services acts. Most of the crimes are considered felonies and carry a fine and jail time of 1 year or more. For example, Missouri's laws rate the abuse in degrees depending on the type of harm caused to the elder. Missouri's laws list who is under a legal duty to report abuse or suspected abuse, including adult day care workers, Christian Science practitioners, embalmers, chiropractors, coroner, and probation or parole officers [10]. When there is evidence of suspicious or questionable financial transactions, the State's Attorney's office should be contacted immediately for more information and investigation. Civil cases are a bit easier to maintain and to prove for several reasons: (1) It is at the discretion of the plaintiff-elder whether to sue or not, (2) there is the potential for financial recovery that is missing from criminal cases, and (3) the burden of proof is lower for civil cases (preponderance of the evidence) than for criminal cases (beyond a reasonable doubt).

Elder law

An Elder Law attorney is a good point of contact for the health care professional who suspects financial abuse. By virtue of the fact the Elder Law attorney works with seniors on more or less a full-time basis, he or she is more attuned to the nuances of the elder population and is usually more patient in dealing with the elder victim. Often, the elder may feel more comfortable speaking with an Elder Law attorney who, with appropriate questions asked in a sympathetic and nonjudgmental manner, may have greater success in uncovering details of potentially abusive acts.

Elder Law is a distinct area of practice defined not so much by the legal issues as it is by the type of client. Like gerontology in medicine, familiarity with general areas of practice is important to the Elder Law attorney, but it is the adaptation of general practice concepts to the senior client that is key and makes the practice area unique. Given the usual unpredictability and rapid pace of changes within state and federal laws, a general practitioner or one who dabbles in the area will have a hard time keeping up with the shifting landscape of Elder Law. An attorney who focuses his practice in Elder Law will likely be current to better represent his elder clients and their families while serving as a reliable resource for other professionals.

An Elder Law attorney is in the unique position of having knowledge of legal issues and a basic working knowledge of the various medical conditions affecting his clients. This basic knowledge clues the Elder Law attorney in to physical or psychologic signs of abuse of all types that may appear during the course of an appointment interview. Assessing capacity of the elder, for example, is an important part of the client interview. Although an Elder Law attorney does not perform medical capacity examinations, simple mental tests can reveal whether the elder client is able to understand and execute documents. Improperly executed documents or an incapacitated client may be key ingredients to a financial abuse case. If presented with an obviously altered Power of Attorney giving unusual or questionable authority to a caregiver, an Elder Law attorney familiar with the Durable Power of Attorney documents generally used in his state or locale may be quick to find evidence of financial exploitation.

Health care professionals might take a page from the Elder Law attorney's play book when it comes to interviewing patients who may be victims of any abuse, including financial exploitation. Attorneys generally meet with the elder without any family members or caregivers in the room to verify the elder's wishes and elicit their concerns. Confidentiality is paramount along with the assurance that information will not be divulged without the senior's permission. The elder must be assured that, as the client, he/she is in control. Once the senior is back in the presence of the suspected abuser, the practitioner should be alert to signs of fear, excessive deference to the suspected abuser, or anxiety. It is important the elder be discouraged from rationalizing or accepting the abusive behavior. Acceptance of abusive behavior means the elder will not report it and that the abuser will continue on with the behavior.

Medical aspects

There may be few opportunities within the institutional or hospital setting for a health care professional to notice financial abuse. It is likely to be more apparent in the office or home setting.

In the office, a practitioner may notice certain indicators of financial abuse. For example, the patient might be inappropriately dressed for the season (shirt sleeves in very cold weather) or complains of "no money" or decreased funds available to him. The elder patient may be accompanied by a caregiver or family member who seems overly protective or refuses to allow the elder to speak for himself. There may be long periods of time between office visits. The elder's level of care may decrease significantly or may not be commensurate with the elder's demonstrated ability to pay for such care in the past.

The home setting may provide the health care professional with the best opportunities for discovering financial abuse. Utilities may be shut off, excessive numbers of magazines not related to the patient's life or interests, or the existence of reading material in the home of a blind or sight-compromised patient should raise suspicions. The lack of food in sufficient amounts or types may be a clue that money is not available to the elder and possibly diverted away. These signs may indicate other forms of abuse as well, so the home health care professional should be aware of these observations.

Awareness of the possibility of abuse is the first step for health care professionals. Evaluation, treatment, and prevention of future episodes are appropriate follow-up steps.

Development of detecting and screening protocol

Development of a protocol useful to health care professionals in handling incidents of financial elder abuse is important. Elements of a detection and screening program should include the following.

Detection

Identification of Highest Risk Situations Likely to Lead to Elder Abuse, using the acronym SAVED, includes identifying the following [15]:

- Stress/social isolation
- Alcohol/other drug abuse
- Violent history
- Emotional or psychiatric illness
- Dependency, dynamic of the family

Table 1
Evaluation decisions

Physical abuse/medical response	Financial abuse response
Subjective	Subjective
Statements of patient: "I am dizzy and hurt in my stomach."	Statements by elder: "My son stole everything I own; I haven't got a dime"; apparent deprivation of goods and services; exacerbation of existing conditions
Objective	
Injury evidenced by physical signs and symptoms (bruising, burns, pain, swelling, etc.), the presence of obvious physical injuries, or injuries revealed upon examination and testing	Objective
	Evidence of unusual banking activity, existence of unpaid bills, low bank balance
Assessment	Assessment
Emergency care required for physical corresponding medical treatments for injuries, conditions discovered	Interrupt abuser's ability to continue harmful practices; prevent further "bleeding"of assets; financial abuse is often chronic and subtle, involves "poisonous" relationships
Plan/treatment	Plan/treatment
Order appropriate lab tests and discharge when stable with instructions to follow up as necessary.	Remove elder from abusive situation; involve nurses and ancillary personnel such as social workers, attorneys, community resources, advocacy agencies in finding, correcting; eliminate opportunities for abuse; long-term follow-up care should be included in plans.

Evaluation

A diagnostic decision tree is used to evaluate physical signs and symptoms when a patient presents for treatment. A similar decision tree can be used to evaluate elder financial abuse. Abuse should be considered if there are warning signs or suspicious signs and symptoms lacking any other explanation. Table 1 presents a side-by-side comparison of evaluation decisions that tracks how the process can proceed. As with all forms of abuse, it is important to remember that the elder may not be forthcoming with information or may deny that there is abusive treatment.

Barriers to identification

The victim's unwillingness or inability to cooperate with those in a position to help is not the only reason financial abuse is under-reported or misdiagnosed. It is sometimes the health care professional's problem as well. Various personal barriers may include the following:

- Frustration with or inability to relate to elders
- Difficulty with interpretation of subtle signs of abuse that could indicate other problems (eg, social withdrawal, poor hygiene)
- Lack of routine for detection and screening
- Inadequate social services available for follow-up
- Lack of coordination between health care providers and social/community/ governmental agencies

Documentation

Once identified, accurate and sufficiently detailed documentation is important to help avoid misdiagnosis, develop profiles and patterns of behavior for future identification of abuse, and prepare safe discharge plans.

Interview the suspected abuser

- Interview the elder separately from the suspected abuser
- Note inconsistencies in stories or event description as provided by each party
- Note nonverbal cues throughout entire interview but especially when elder and suspected abuser are together
- Compare the elder's demeanor when alone and with suspected abuser, documenting verbal and nonverbal cues

General characteristics of abusers

The health care professional should be familiar with the general characteristics of an elder abuser and make appropriate notations.

- The abuser may be harsh or aggressive toward the elder.
- The elder may be prevented or discouraged from speaking to the health care professional; there may be evidence of intimidation.
- The abuser may have isolated the elder from family members or social activities.
- There may be inconsistent descriptions of events and actions by the abuser when recounting activities to different interviewers or by the elder when her story does not match the physical evidence.
- The abuser may be dependent on the elder for financial support.

Reporting

Accurate documentation and reporting are keys to the development of sufficient and meaningful legal remedies and useful medical treatments. Ethical considerations of reporting any type of abuse against the elder's will or returning the elder to the abusive environment are major concerns of those responsible for reporting elder abuse. Also, because the elder is an adult and presumably capable of making decisions about his care, he has the right to refuse services or care. The health care professional cannot hospitalize the elder on suspicions of elder abuse if the elder protests.

Each state has its own laws in place for addressing elder abuse. These laws are usually found in the Adult Protection Services (APS) statutes. The national hotline for locating safe, reputable services and housing for elders is 1-800-677-1116. If an emergency exists, it is appropriate to call the local 911 services for assistance.

It is a legal duty of health care professional, indeed to report suspicious activity that raises a "reasonable belief" that an elder has been or is likely to be abused, neglected, or exploited [16]. Health care professionals can be of invaluable assistance to Elder Law attorneys by creating detailed clinical notes covering the following ares:

- Relevant history in the elder's own words (helpful, but not a requirement) using broad questions to define the potential type(s) of abuse, such as
  Do you support anyone financially?
  Have you noticed anything missing lately?
  Have you signed any legal papers recently?
  Have you signed several blank checks all at once and then given them to someone to use to pay your bills?
  Who pays your bills?

- Health questions that are part of a typical patient assessment interview, including
  Past medical history
  Physical complaints
  Habits, social activities
  Family members (live-in, living elsewhere)/relationships, significant others
  Caregivers (live-in, come-and-go)
- Physical examination is helpful, including:
  Health conditions that may mimic abuse to rule out suspected abuse
  Recurrent or untreated conditions (eg, due to unfilled prescriptions)
- Psychologic evaluation may reveal existence of
  Tendencies toward or actual existence of psychiatric disorders
  Dementia (Alzheimer's and non-Alzheimer's-type)
  Lack of capacity

Development of safe discharge plan

It is important to remove the elder from the situation that lead to the abuse in the first place if at all possible. Closure of accounts in joint names of the elder victim and the abuser is necessary to interrupt access and to the elder's funds. If the elder agrees, use a geriatric case manager or other professional for oversight and management of the elder's funds and bill-paying.

Follow-up

Short-term and long-term follow-up is necessary to prevent the abuser from coming back into the elder's life or re-establishing a fiduciary relationship with the victim. The elder should be evaluated on a continuous basis in the office and at the home (a personal residence or a facility). Social Services or the Visiting Nurses Association should follow up as well to make any other needed recommendations for assistance, such as a geriatric case manager. On-going follow-up also reminds the elder to be on the look-out for scams or other financial exploitation.

Prevention

As with most forms of abuse, the best offense is an effective defense: Prevent the abuse before it happens by decreasing the opportunities for exploitation. Virtually anyone who has contact with elders, and even elders themselves, can help prevent financial abuse. Without clearcut symptoms to be aware of, the elder may not seem to be in any obvious harm. There are, however, several factors common to all abuse cases, including financial abuse.

- A trusting relationship in which the elder feels comfortable confiding in the potential abuser
- The abuser's motivation to abuse being due to real or perceived financial need
- Clear and open opportunities to steal from or exploit the elder without being caught

Interruption at any of these points prevents or at least slow down the continued actions of an abuser. If immediate intervention is necessary, it is important to ascertain whether the abuser has access to the elder's funds. Steps should be taken to freeze bank or other financial accounts to prevent further activity on the account. Remove any joint account holders' name(s), especially if the name has recently been added or is that of someone not normally expected to be a joint account holder. Replace the suspected abuser's name with someone neutral, such as a bonded professional or a family member known to be a nonabusive person. A new account should be opened into which existing funds or direct deposit funds can be placed. Checks should be kept in a safe place, not easily accessed without the elder's permission. Blank checks should not be signed individually or several at a time and then given to a third party to use. Personal identification numbers, Social Security numbers, and similar security information for access to ATMs or other financial resources should not be freely shared or divulged.

Credit card use should be kept to a minimum, and the credit limit should be kept low. If the card is lost or stolen, it is easier to replace or cancel one versus many cards. Restriction of charges to one card allows for easier tracking of purchases. A low limit discourages or prevents the accumulation of a large debt. An attempt to make a large purchase and a low limit may trigger an inquiry by the issuing credit card company and the refusal of authorization for the purchase.

With all financial transactions, if fraud or theft is suspected, stop payment on the checks and close the account as soon as possible. Bank and other financial statements should be reviewed periodically to pick up any changes in the usual flow of banking activity.

As the elder's advocate, an Elder Law attorney should be consulted to do several things on behalf of an abused elder. A restraining order can be sought against the alleged abuser to keep him away from the elder or the elder's funds. All legal documents should be checked for validity. It may be necessary to have new Powers of Attorney drafted and signed by the victim if he/she is able to do so. If the elder does not have the mental capacity to understand the purpose of the Power of Attorney document and that he/she is giving someone else the right to act on his/her behalf, guardianship or conservatorship is necessary to protect the elder's funds. When appointing an individual to manage the affairs of another via a court-order, some states use the designation of "Guardian of the Estate" (for financial affairs) or "Guardian of the Person" (for health care and other personal decision-making). Other states use the title "Conservator" for the appointee who manages financial decision-making for the incapacitated person. A temporary guardian appointment may be obtained relatively quickly as long as a plenary or full guardianship appointment is sought shortly thereafter. If real property is at risk of being sold, a lis pendens action may be filed (lis pendens literally means "a pending law suit" [8]), putting anyone doing a title search on notice there is litigation pending and thereby halting the transaction or putting it on hold.

Newly executed Powers of Attorney documents should be carefully and closely scrutinized. If there are suspicions, tell the presenter-agent of a questionable Power of Attorney document that a call to the elder is necessary to verify the agent's status.

If possible, the elder and her agents pursuant to the Powers of Attorney for Health Care and Property (separate documents, generally) should get to know their health care providers and financial advisors/bankers. If a professional knows that an elderly account holder does not often get out or is unable to sign her name, even slight increases in bank account use may be detected and investigated quicker than if the account holder was not so familiar.

Be leery of Trust or Estate Planning seminars that promise low or no-cost document services. The consumer usually gets what he pays for in that case—nothing. Consult an Elder Law or Estate Planning attorney if a plan is needed or if an existing plan should be reviewed or updated.

Other important documents should be reviewed. Life insurance policies may have been changed to name the abuser as beneficiary. Retirement and "Pay On Death" accounts may have been changed by the abuser naming himself as beneficiary. An attorney should be consulted about any changes made to an elder's Will or Trust or other estate-related document. Often, the drafting attorney keeps the original or a signed copy of the document on file, which can be reviewed for discrepancies or alterations. Health care billing statements should be reviewed before payment. Charges for services not ordered or performed can signal financial abuse.

Medicare and Medicaid (Medi-Cal in California) numbers (usually Social Security numbers) should never be given out in situations involving "free" health care services or in unusual situations involving health care professionals. A twist on the home improvement scam is the "Let us check the 'health' of your Medicare benefits to be sure you are fully covered. Now, just fill in this form with your Social Security number...." scam.

Protect credit card numbers and Social Security numbers at all times. The elder should not give out any personally identifying information over the telephone or Internet, especially when the elder did not initiate the contact. Unknown religions or charitable organizations can sound worthwhile to vulnerable elders (or anyone).

A mail box rented at the post office for receipt of mail makes it less likely the elder's mail will be diverted or intercepted.

Once the financial abuse/exploitation has been detected and stopped, there are ways to prevent its recurrence.

- A commercial service or geriatric care manager can be hired to pay bills and oversee the running of the elder's household and caregivers. Daily Money Management programs are few in number but are becoming more popular by offering help with bill paying, check preparation, management of household expenses and employees (including payroll), preparation of income tax returns, and so forth [17].
- Designate a Representative Payee for government benefits, including Social Security, VA benefits, or Railroad Retirement benefits. A "Rep. Payee" may be designated on a form available from the government office issuing the benefits.
- Direct deposit of checks. In addition to naming a Representative Payee, government and any income checks should be directly deposited into the elder's bank account to remove the possibility of interception from a third party.

State and federal response

Elder financial abuse is a local and a national problem; anywhere there is an elder, there is the potential for abuse.

Federal laws

There are no federally funded programs specifically geared toward the protection of victims of elder abuse, although there are such programs for domestic violence and child abuse. There is federal level legislation that targets prevention of elder abuse, neglect, and exploitation.

The Administration on Aging, part of the federal Department of Health and Human Services, is responsible for Administration of the Older Americans Act Title VII entitled "Vulnerable Elder Rights Protection" [18]. This legislation includes provisions for long-term care ombudsman programs, public education, and legal assistance program development at the state level. With a relatively small budget of just over $5 million, the Act is underfunded, yet it is a vital source of information and is a funding source for the National Center on Elder Abuse [19].

The NCEA is a great resource for all things related to elder abuse. There is a wealth of state-specific information as well. The site is not exhaustive of all legislative and legal information. Individual states may have additional remedies within domestic or family violence acts, guardianship/conservatorship statutes, and the laws relating to durable powers of attorney. The regulations and policies of state departments on aging should be reviewed for relevant elder abuse information.

Because Medicaid fraud is a form of financial abuse, the federal government polices health care providers or the system through Fraud Control Systems. The

Office of Inspector General Annual Report on State Medicaid Fraud Control Units for fiscal year 2003 (October 1, 2002 to September 30, 2003) [20] revealed that 47 states and the District of Columbia participated in the Medicaid Fraud Control Grant Program. The mission of this program is to investigate and prosecute Medicaid provider fraud and patient abuse and neglect. Most Medicaid Fraud Control Units are part of the Office of States Attorney General or part of another state agency related to elder services. According to this report, during 2003, $268 million was recovered in court-ordered restitutions, fines, civil settlements, and penalties; 1096 convictions were obtained; 538 individuals and entities were excluded from participating in the Medicare/medicaid programs; and 5570 patient abuse and neglect cases were opened over the course of the year [20].

The Health Insurance Portability and Accountability Act established a national health care fraud and abuse control program. The Attorney General and the Secretary of Health and Human Services are responsible for coordination of federal, state, and local law enforcement programs aimed at identifying and prosecuting health care fraud. The program addresses fraud and abuse against all levels of health care providers including Certified Nurse Assistants, Dentists, Billing Services, Durable Medical Equipment Companies, Home Health Care Services, Hospitals, Laboratories, Nurses, Nursing homes, Optometrists, Ortho-dontist (juvenile cases of abuse), Pharmacies, Physicians, Psychologists, Trans-portation Services, and others [21].

State laws

There is considerably more elder abuse prevention legislation at the state level. All 50 states and the District of Columbia have laws addressing various aspects of reporting and preventing elder abuse. All states have enacted specific elder-related APS acts and long-term care ombudsman programs. Only 13 states, not including the District of Columbia, have enacted Institutional Abuse Legis-lation (aimed at nursing homes, assisted living facilities, and board and care homes) [16].

There is little state legislation specifically addressing elder financial abuse, and there is great variability among the legislation that does exist. Illinois, for example, has nine general elder abuse legislative programs, but only one addresses financial abuse. This state legislation was recently strengthened when the Illinois governor signed legislation requiring the Office of Banks and Real Estate to work with the Department of Aging in encouraging all Illinois banks and financial institutions to participate in training their employees to identify and prevent different forms of financial abuse. Financial abuse accounted for 55% of all cases of elder abuse in the state of Illinois in 2003 [22]. Illinois' elder abuse laws require reporting by certain professionals, encourage reports by the public, and provide immunity from liability or professional disciplinary action for those who make a good faith abuse report [22]. A program entitled "B*SAFE" (Bankers and Seniors against Financial Exploitation) is administered through the

Department of Aging and provides money management services for elders who have been victimized by financial exploitation [22]. California, on the other hand, has 29 elder abuse-related state law programs, and at least six of those programs are specific to elder financial exploitation prevention. There is no uniformity among the states.

In all cases, federal or state, when financial or any type of abuse is suspected, the reporter is urged to call the state abuse hotline. In an emergency, the police should be called. The state hotline can be found in the phone book or by calling the national toll-free number that locates a dedicated toll-free number for out-of-state callers. A list of state hotlines is available at wwww.elderabusecenter.org (click on the State Hot Lines tab).

Summary

Financial exploitation is the most common form of elder abuse, but it is the probably the most subtle and degrading. Without obvious physical signs that immediately raise suspicions, financial abuse is tough to diagnose on the first or even after several encounters with the elder.

Prevention is the key to reducing the incidence of this type of abuse. Elders should be encouraged to relate suspicions about questionable activities. Bank accounts and other financial sources should be protected from access by third parties without the account holder's permission. Legal documents should be protected from alteration by someone other than an attorney. Legal action is a possible reactive measure.

Public education is the strongest medicine in these cases. Financial abuse is part of a larger problem of generally negative attitudes toward the elderly and the perception that any type of abuse is a private family problem to be kept behind closed doors. Financial exploitation may not leave physical scars, but the emotional hurt may last a long time, especially if the abuser has robbed a senior of hard-earned funds or the only means of support.

Appendix A

Internet resources: financial exploitation and fraud

This is not an exhaustive list; it is representative of the large amount of Internet information available.

California Community Partnership for the Prevention of Financial Abuse: www.bewiseonline.org/index.shtml
Clergy Against Senior Exploitation (CASE): www.denverda.org (Colorado)
Virginia TRIAD Central Office, Office of the Attorney General: www.vaag. com/Protecting/Triad/fraudstats.htm

Financial crimes against the elderly from the US Department of Justice: www.cops.usdoj.gov

US Postal Service and Inspection Service "Senior Fraud Prevention": www.usps.gov at the tab "Office of Inspector General" Financial Exploitation of Elders (National Center for Victims of Crime): www.ncvc.org

US Administration of Aging: www.aoa.gov

US Department of Justice at the Office for Victims of Crime: www.ojp.usdoj.gov/ovc.welcome.html

Elder Abuse Center: www.elderabusecenter.org. Brochure describing financial abuse, signs, and symptoms, etc.: www.co.san-bernardino.ca.us/brochures/docs/105.pdf

Federal Trade Commission and AARP publications describing Alternatives to Guardianship and Money Management Programs: www.ftc.gov/bcp/conline/pubs/services/apact/apact01.htm www.ftc.gov/bcp/conline/pubs/services/apact/apact02.htm

References

[1] The National Center on Elder Abuse. The major areas of elder abuse include physical, sexual, emotional or psychological, neglect, self-neglect, financial or material exploitation. The basics: financial or material exploitation. Available at: www.elderabusecenter.org/default.cfm?p=basics.cfm. Accessed November 6, 2004.

[2] Thomas C. The first national study of elder abuse and neglect: contrast with results from other studies. J Elder Abuse Negl 2000;12:1–14.

[3] Pillemer K, Finkelhor D. Mistreatment Prevalence Study (aka the prevalence of elder abuse: a random sample survey). Gerontology 1988;28:51–7.

[4] The National Elder Abuse Incidence Study. Washington, DC: US Dept. of Health and Human Services, Administration for Children and Families, Administration of Aging; 1998.

[5] Administration on Aging. Elder rights & resources: elder abuse. Available at: www.aoa.dhhs.gov/eldfam/elder_rights/Elder_Abuse/Elder_Abuse.asp. Accessed October 6, 2004.

[6] What is elder abuse. The Elder Abuse Center. Available at www.elderabusecenter.org/basic/indez.html. Accessed October 5, 2004.

[7] Elder abuse: types, signs, symptoms, causes, and help. Available at: www.helpguide.org./mental/elder_abuse_physical_emotional_sexual_neglect.htm. Accessed October 6, 2004.

[8] Black HL, Black HC. Black's Law dictionary. 6th edition. St. Paul (MN): West Publishing Company; 1990.

[9] The National Center on Elder Abuse. Is elder abuse a crime? Available at: www.elderabusecenter.org/print_page.cfm?p=iselderabuseacrime.cfm. Accessed October 5, 2004.

[10] Missouri stat 565.180 RSMO.

[11] Missouri stat 660.250 RSMO et seq.

[12] Missouri stat 660.300 RSMO et seq.

[13] Missouri stat 558.011RSMO.

[14] Missouri stat 565.188 RSMO.

[15] Woolard R, Bernstein E. Elder abuse. In: Society for Academic Emergency Medicine. Available at: www.saem.org/inform/eldabuse.htm. Accessed October 5, 2004.

[16] American Bar Association Commission on Problems of the Elderly. Elder abuse laws. Available at: www.elderabusecenter.org/laws/index,html. Accessed October 5, 2004.

[17] Nerenberg L. Daily money management programs; a protection against elder abuse. San Francisco: Institute on Aging; 2003.

[18] 42 U.S.C. §3058a, et seq.

[19] The National Center on Elder Abuse. Available at: wwwelderabusecenter.org/print_page. cfm?p=statelaws.cfm. Accessed November 6, 2004.

[20] Medicaid Fraud Control Units (MFCU) HHS-OIG Publications. Available at: www.oig.dhhs.gov/ Publications/docs/mcfu/MCFU2003.pdf. Accessed October 5, 2004.

[21] Administration on Aging. Available at: www.aoa.dhhs.gov. Accessed October 6, 2004.

[22] Blagojevich signs law to strengthen state protection of elder rights. Available at: www.illinois. gov/PressReleases/PrintPressRelease.cfm?subjectID=3&RecNum=32. Accessed October 5, 2004.

ELSEVIER
SAUNDERS

CLINICS IN
GERIATRIC
MEDICINE

Clin Geriatr Med 21 (2005) 383–398

The Legal and Governmental Response to Domestic Elder Abuse

Ray J. Koenig III, JD[a],*, Cameron R. DeGuerre[a,b]

[a]Peck, Bloom, Austriaco & Mitchell, LLC, 105 West Adams Street, 31st Floor,
Chicago, IL 60603, USA
[b]DePaul University College of Law, 25 East Jackson Boulevard, Chicago, IL 60604, USA

Lillian is an 83-year-ld California resident who lives with her son, Richard. Richard has a history of untreated substance abuse. During an alcohol-induced rampage, Richard hit Lillian over the head with beer bottles, struck her across the face, pushed her onto the floor, and threatened her life. He spent all of their money on alcohol, denying her adequate nutrition.

Glenda, a 72-year-old woman, lives with her mentally ill daughter, Sara. Sara ridicules her mother by laughing at her when she is speaking and telling Glenda that she is ruining her life. She constantly rearranges the furniture and makes fun of Glenda when she becomes disoriented. Sara's constant practical jokes and ill-tempered behavior leaves Glenda feeling lonely, isolated, and worthless.

Frank is an 84-year-old retired veteran who lives alone in a one-bedroom apartment in a large residential complex. Frank's neighbor, Susan, began dropping by on the weekends for friendly chats. Frank enjoyed their time together, and, eventually, Susan was visiting four or five times per week. They formed a close, trusting relationship. During one of their visits, Susan became visibly upset and told Frank about a serious financial situation that caused her to max out several of her credit cards. Her total debt amounted to $20,000. She told Frank that she would have to move to a cheaper apartment unless she could find a way to pay off part of her debt. Desperate to keep his new friend, Frank

---

Although elder abuse is prevalent in domestic and institutional settings, this article is limited to the legal and governmental response to domestic elder abuse. There are a variety of federal and state laws targeting abuse in institutional settings; however, analysis of these laws should be addressed in a separate article.

* Corresponding author.
E-mail address: rkoenig@peckbloom.com (R.J. Koenig III).

loaned Susan $10,000 to pay off a portion of her debt. Susan cashed the check, moved out of her apartment, and never spoke to Frank again.

Jerry, a 72-year-old Iowa native, lives with his son Bill, his daughter-in-law Beth, and their three children. Jerry is wheelchair bound and requires assistance with his daily activities. Bill is a traveling salesman and is constantly out of town on business-related trips. When Bill is out of town, Beth often overlooks Jerry's needs in a struggle to take care of her home and family. During these times, Jerry misses meals and medication and often goes unbathed.

John is a 68-year-old Arkansas resident who lives alone in a small, rural community. John suffers from early stage Alzheimer disease. His family lives across the country and has tried on several occasions to convince him to move into an assisted living community. All attempts were unsuccessful. Three months ago, his daughter went to visit him in an effort to convince him to hire a caregiver. She was distraught when she found her father sitting alone in his house, physically weak and covered in filth. The house was filled with garbage and half-eaten meals and was infested with roaches.

Some of the instances of elder abuse and neglect described above may seem extreme, but they are not uncommon. The purpose of this article is to create a general understanding of domestic elder abuse, highlight its prevalence, and analyze the legal response on the federal and state levels to this serious problem.

The prevalence of elder abuse

Although the number of elder abuse and neglect cases per year cannot be determined, in 1981 the United States Congress House Select Committee of Aging issued a report estimating that over 1,000,000 elderly Americans annually are victims of physical, emotional, and financial abuse by their loved ones [1]. The report also highlighted the hidden nature of elder abuse: Only one out of every six victims is likely to report mistreatment to the appropriate legal authorities. The Committee recommended that the States enact statutes, modeled after recent child abuse legislation, designating state agencies to identify and assist elder abuse victims. Congress was urged to enact legislation to provide financial assistance to the states in support of these programs [1].

Ten years later, the same Committee issued a follow-up report, *Elder Abuse: A Decade of Shame and Inaction*. The congressional findings indicated that the situation had worsened. The second report concluded that every year 5% of the nation's elderly population (more than 1,500,000 elderly persons) annually are victims of physical, psychological, and financial exploitation [2].

The Committee determined that elder abuse cases are far less likely than child abuse cases to be reported to local authorities. Although one out of every three child abuse cases was reported in 1989, only one out of eight elder abuse cases came to the attention of local authorities [2,3]. The Committee determined that funding to investigate and rectify such incidents was disproportionate to the resources used to investigate child abuse. For example, in 1989, $45.03 was spent per state child resident for protective services, whereas only $3.80 was spent per state elder resident for the same services [2]. Without federal financial assistance, the states are hard pressed to implement the new social services. Additionally, although four fifths of the states had created mandatory reporting laws between 1981 and 1990, state implementation and enforcement of the laws await federal financial assistance [2].

Population of older Americans

The importance of calling national attention to elder abuse cannot be overstated. Demographics indicate the increasing need for public attention in the area. Older Americans comprise the fastest growing segment of the United States population [4–6]. According to the United States Census Bureau, in 1994 people 65 years of age and older accounted for 12.8% of the United States population [4]. By the year 2020, it is estimated that this group will increase by 3.8%. In the year 2050, older Americans may account for 20% of the population [7].

Although older Americans constitute the fastest growing segment of the nation's population, governmental interest in identifying and solving the problems of the elderly population has developed at a much slower pace [5]. Congressional and scholarly research estimates that between one and two million instances of abuse occur per year [2]. Few instances are reported to state agencies. Of those reported, the scarcity of resources available to state agencies allows minimal action at best [2,8].

Legal definitions of abuse and neglect

Elder abuse can generally be described as sustained physical or psychologic assault of an older person. Elder abuse can be distinguished from ordinary criminal behavior because it usually does not consist of a single incident of conduct. Rather, it usually consists of repetitive instances of misconduct [9]. Almost all abuse victims have an ongoing relationship with their abuser. Abuse is usually inflicted by an elder's caregiver but is not necessarily isolated to those living with the abused elder [9].

The five main types of elder mistreatment are physical abuse, psychological abuse, financial exploitation, neglect, and self-neglect [10]. No single definition encompasses all forms of mistreatment. Analysis of publications by federal agencies dedicated to elder abuse supplies the following general definitions of abuse:

• Physical abuse involves threatening actions that result in physical injury, pain, or impairment [11]. The abuse can be active (striking the victim) or passive (withholding necessary medication) but need not involve assault. Common examples include hitting, shoving, physically restraining another, and sexually assaulting or molesting an elderly individual [10,12]. Lillian's story at the beginning of this article represents an example of physical abuse.

- Psychological abuse includes verbal or nonverbal acts that result in severe mental anguish to another [11]. The abuse ranges from name-calling to dehumanizing remarks made with the intention to exhaust an individual's self-worth. Psychological abuse causes the abused elder to suffer from shame, humiliation, and embarrassment [10,12]. An example of psychological abuse is Glenda, noted at the beginning of this article.
- Financial exploitation is theft or conversion of an elderly individual's property or assets [11]. It can range from expropriating or appropriating an elder's funds to inducing them to sign documents that substantially diminish their legal control over assets or transfer such authority to another. Financial exploitation is commonly accompanied by physical or psychologic abuse [10,12]. The relationship between Frank and Susan, discussed at the beginning of this article, illustrates a form of financial exploitation.
- Neglect is the failure to fulfill a care-taking obligation that is necessary to the good health and overall well-being of the elderly individual [11]. It can be active or passive. Active neglect is determined by the caretaker's volition (ie, whether the caretaker actions are intentional). Passive neglect may be the result of mere ignorance. For example, a caretaker's failure to understand the implications of a serious medical illness may cause him or her to be apathetic in filling prescription medications for the elderly individual. This may result in rapid development of illness and may cause unnecessary suffering by the elderly individual [10,12]. Jerry's situation, described at the beginning of this article, provides an example of passive neglect.
- Self-neglect includes behaviors by an elderly person that threaten his or her safety or well-being. These may include the older person's refusal to provide herself with life necessities such as food, water, clothing, personal hygiene, medication, and shelter. The decision to withhold such necessities (by a competent elderly individual) for whatever reason is included in the definition of self-neglect. Self-neglect may constitute elder abuse if perpetrated by an individual whose relationship with the older adult (eg, spousal relationship, duty pursuant to a contract, or assumed caregiving role) requires action to rectify the individual's self-destructive behavior. In such a case, the law mandates a duty to act, the failure of which is legally actionable [10,12]. John's story, described at the beginning of this article, provides an example of self-neglect.

The legal response to abuse and neglect

The law has primarily responded to elder abuse and mistreatment in three ways: through the use of (1) legal mandates, (2) criminal laws, and (3) community-based education [5]. Legal mandates are implemented through state statutes and require professionals and other designated individuals to report reasonably suspected instances of abuse to the appropriate state agency. Criminal laws outlaw certain types of behavior as inappropriate mistreatment and prescribe punishments accordingly. Educational programs are given at the local level in which small, independent agencies strive to promote general awareness in the community regarding the pervasiveness of the problem, indications of abuse, and preventative techniques [5].

Elder abuse is among the most recent forms of domestic violence to command public attention. Although reports of "granny bashing" were disseminated in Great Britain during the early 1970s, studies indicating that elder abuse was a national problem in the United States did not appear until the end of that decade [5]. Despite the increase in research, there are far fewer comprehensive studies dedicated to elder abuse than there are for child and spousal abuse [13].

The federal government's response to domestic elder abuse

Although elder abuse was identified by Congress as a national problem in the late 1970s and subsequently addressed in federal legislation, there is no federal statute specifically dedicated to preventing the mistreatment of elderly persons similar to those targeted at child abuse and domestic violence. Amendments to the Older Americans Act of 1965, enacted in 1992, provided definitions of elder abuse and further authorized funding for elder abuse awareness, training, and coordination activities but provided only minimal funds to adult protective services or shelters [12,14]. Based on a study conducted by the National Center on Elder Abuse (NCEA) in the year 2000, the Older Americans Act provided an average of $59,795 in funding to seven states. Five states reportedly received no funding pursuant to grants authorized by the Older Americans Act [8]. The other 42 states[1] did not respond to questions regarding federal funding.

In 1974, Title XX of the Social Security Act mandated the states to provide services to meet the social, psychologic, medical, and legal needs of people with physical and mental disabilities who were at risk of being neglected or exploited or who were unable to manage their own affairs [15]. The act provides Social Service Block Grants to the states. These programs did not develop due to widespread criticism that they were costly and ineffective and that they potentially infringed on civil rights. Some opponents of the act argued that the stigma associated with public welfare would be more prejudicial than helpful. As a result, Title XX federal block grants decreased dramatically during the 1980s [5].

In 1981, the Select Committee on Aging of the United States House of Representatives issued a report, *Elder Abuse: An Examination of a Hidden Problem*, that drew national attention to elder abuse and mistreatment. This report attempted to define elder abuse and determine its prevalence among the popu-

---

[1] The sample for the NCEA study included all 50 states, the District of Columbia, and Guam. Louisiana and Oregon had two separate statutes addressing adult protective service programs and therefore are counted twice.

lation. It concluded that elder abuse is a hidden yet national problem crossing all segments of the population [1]. It is one of the few areas in which barriers such as race, ethnicity, and socio-economic status have minimal effect [5,9,13].

Little federal action followed the 1981 report. The Elder Abuse Treatment & Prevention Act was introduced in the 96th Congress in 1991 and in subsequent sessions of Congress but never passed [5]. No federal policy or financing has been initiated to address noninstitutionalized elderly persons living in the community.

Funding from federal block grants continues to be minimal. In the year 2000, it was reported that only 13 states received funding from the Social Service Block Grants. This has caused the states to use general funds to finance state services directed toward elder abuse victims [8].

The Proposed Elder Justice Act of 2003, formerly the Elder Justice Act of 2002, may provide solutions by filling in the gaps of current federal laws. If passed, the act would provide federal resources to support state and community efforts to fight elder abuse. It proposes the creation of the following offices: (1) the Office of Elder Justice in the Department of Health and Human Services and a companion office in the Department of Justice, which would provide programmatic, grant-making, policy, and technical assistance functions relating to elder justice; and (2) a federal Coordinating Council to coordinate the activities of all relevant federal agencies, state, community, and private not-for-profit entities [16,17].

The primary elements of the act consist of the following [16,17]:

- To increase knowledge and support based on projects regarding elder abuse
- To develop data about forensic markers and methodologies
- To create victim's assistance safe havens and support for elders at risk of abuse
- To increase prosecution of elder abuse cases
- To create the National Justice Library of Technical Assistance and Promising Practice Materials, which would research topics regarding elder abuse and provide training information
- To grant state funds to streamline a reporting system for elder abuse cases
- To create special programs for underserved populations
- To publish model state laws and practices to facilitate a uniform policy on elder abuse
- To increase security, collaboration, and consumer information in long-term care for elders
- To maintain consistent funding and national coordination for adult protective services

The states' responses to domestic elder abuse

The states' responses to the 1981 House Select Committee Report were remarkably different from the federal government's response. Until 1977, no state had a statute specifically aimed at protecting the elderly population. By 1985, anticipating federal financial assistance, over 44 states had enacted such legislation [2,5]. Presently, all 50 states have statutes aimed at protecting the elderly population [8]. State legislation for elder abuse is modeled after child abuse and domestic violence statutes and typically includes two components: (1) coordinated provisions of services for elders determined to be susceptible to some form of abuse and (2) provisions providing state agencies with actual or potential power to intervene and protect endangered adults. State statutes have been the primary engine for combating elder abuse. This is most often seen through the implementation of adult protective services [10].

Adult protective services target elderly individuals or people with disabilities who are in danger of being mistreated or neglected and are unable to protect themselves due to isolation or vulnerability [8]. Because there is minimal federal funding provided to some states' adult protective services, most states have been forced to develop individual programs and re-allocate funding formerly used for other state social services [8].

Most state adult protective services are offered to vulnerable adults. A vulnerable adult is commonly defined as a person who is being mistreated or is susceptible to mistreatment and is unable to protect himself as a result of old age or disability [8]. Although many states provide adult protective services regardless of an individual's age, statutes vary. Some states provide services based on the older person's age alone, whereas others provide such services only after an individual has been declared incapacitated or disabled. Others require a combination of the two requirements [8].

Adult protective services

Adult protective services are mandated by state laws and aim to provide a centralized system to (1) receive reports of abuse and neglect, (2) investigate such reports, (3) intervene by providing services to the victims, and (4) deliver services to abused elders with diminished capacity through involuntary intervention [10,18]. In many jurisdictions, adult protective services are authorized to protect victims in institutional settings and those living in the community [10]. Virtually all adult protective service agencies are within a state's department of health and human services agency or similar social service agency [19].

Mandatory reporting laws.   The issue of whether reporting known or suspected incidents of elder mistreatment should be made mandatory by professionals has conjured heated debate among scholars and professionals. Despite considerable arguments against such mandates, virtually every state requires professionals to report suspected or known abuse. However, mandatory reporting laws are not universal, and some states call for voluntary reporting in their statutes [10].

In general, mandatory reporting laws require a wide variety of professionals and other statutorily designated individuals to report known or suspected incidents of elder abuse and mistreatment [19]. Mandatory reporters typically include professionals in the health care and social services fields [6,11]. For example, a typical state statute requires psychologists, nurses, physicians, surgeons, law-enforcement personnel, and members of the clergy to report abuse [6,8,19].

State statutes vary regarding the definitions of protected individuals. Some states protect all "vulnerable," "disabled," or "incapacitated" individuals regardless of age. Others protect such individuals over a designated age, usually 60 or 65 [5].

All states include physical harm and neglect within their definition of abuse. However, for physical harm, some states' definitions require willful infliction of injury or deprivation of necessary care-taking services to constitute abuse [5,20]. Financial exploitation is almost always covered. Self-neglect is included as abuse in over half of the states. Some states include emotional abuse or mental anguish as prohibited conduct. These terms present difficulties in classification and in distinguishing individuals' levels of tolerance for abuse [20]. Sexual abuse is a separate category of abuse in some states, whereas in others it is encompassed in the general definition of abuse [5].

Reports are typically made to state, regional, or local agencies. These generally include a state's social service agency or part of the long-term care ombudsman program [19]. Most statutes designate a time frame in which the professional must report the abuse to a specific agency or authority [21]. Time frames vary from state to state: Some mandate immediate reporting, others permit reports to be submitted within 10 days, and some fail to mention a time frame in which reports must be received [5]. State authorities and agencies designated to receive the reports also vary by state [21]. Health care professionals should consult their state statute to determine the appropriate and required manner of reporting abuse.

The failure to comply with reporting requirements is usually punishable as a misdemeanor. Other punishments include imprisonment and fines. Some state statutes make no mention of a penalty for failure to report. However, most state statutes create liability for the caretaker of an elderly person who willfully commits an abusive act or commits an abusive act by omission. A caretaker is typically defined as an individual or entity that bears responsibility for the vulnerable adult as a result of family relationship, voluntary assumption of a care-taking role, or duty pursuant to a contract [5,20].

Professionals may be hesitant to report abuse, fearing legal action by the alleged abuser if the report is not substantiated by the state's social service agency [5]. In an effort to create an incentive to comply, many states provide some degree of immunity from prosecution and civil lawsuits to professionals who report pursuant to the statutory requirements [11,20]. Although some states grant absolute civil and criminal immunity to reporters, others require that the reporters act in good faith and without malicious intent before invoking protection [20,21]. A few states waive the physician-patient privilege in an effort to alleviate the tension between a physician's duty of confidentially to the patient and an obligation to comply with the law [21].

Advocates of mandatory reporting statutes argue that the laws create heightened awareness of elder abuse among professionals, specifically physicians, who come into close contact with what may otherwise be an isolated older individual [21]. It has been established that more incidents of elder abuse are reported as a result of such laws. A report issued by the National Center on Elder Abuse, *A Response to the Abuse of Vulnerable Adults: The 2000 Survey of State Adult Protective Services*, identified that family members, health care professionals, and social service agency staff reported the most instances of abuse [8]. However, most state statutes mandate a wide range of professionals to report abuse. The study recommended educational programs to increase reporting by professionals such as physicians, law enforcement personnel, members of the clergy, employees of financial institutions, and others who have frequent contact with elderly persons but are currently not reporting instances of abuse [8].

The three main arguments against mandatory reporting laws can be summarized as follows: (1) Mandatory reporting laws are paternalistic and interfere with the elder's right to self-determination, (2) mandatory reporting violates the confidentially requirement inherent in the physician-patient relationship, and (3) mandatory reporting discourages victims from reporting instances of abuse on their own behalf [5].

Advocates of these laws counter with persuasive arguments. Scholars have recognized that mandatory reporting laws were created out of necessity. Due to the lack of federal funding, states were forced to implement a cost-effective response to elder abuse [21]. The close contact between professionals and elders makes professionals primary candidates for identifying and reporting instances of abuse [21]. Professional medical organizations, such as the American Medical Association (AMA), have identified physicians' crucial role in "lessening the prevalence, scope and severity of …elder abuse" [22] and further advocate compliance with "the laws for requiring reporting of suspected cases of abuse" of elderly individuals [23]. An ethics opinion states that physicians "have an obligation to familiarize themselves with protocols for diagnosing and treating abuse" of the elderly [23]. The AMA urges physicians to receive "train[ing] in issues of family and intimate partner violence through undergraduate and graduate medical education as well as continuing professional development" [22].

Involuntary interventions—guardianship proceedings.   Virtually every state's adult protective services law provides a mechanism for involuntary intervention when the elderly individual is incapable of consenting or objects to assistance. Interventions commonly include the appointment of a guardian or conservator and removing the elderly individual from the abusive environment [10]. A guardian is appointed upon the filing of a petition by an interested person or by the disabled person. The court makes a determination of the alleged disabled person's ability to manage his or her personal or financial affairs [20,24].

Many states authorize the use of a limited guardian. In a limited guardianship, the court limits the guardian's authority to matters beyond the ward's ability to decide. This stands in sharp contrast with previous statutes, which allowed only for the appointment of general or plenary guardians and which leave the ward with no ability to make personal or financial decisions on his or her own behalf. The appointment of a plenary guardian is still available and is appropriate if the elderly individual is adjudged totally incapable of managing his or her personal or financial affairs. The flexibility in the statutes allows courts to tailor the guardianship to the individual's specific situation while honoring the individual's rights [20].

Domestic violence legislation

Virtually every state and the District of Columbia have laws aimed at preventing or punishing domestic violence [5]. Domestic violence laws were designed to combat family violence, typically spousal and intimate partner violence, but are an effective tool in the fight against elder abuse [10]. Under a typical domestic violence statute, a judge is authorized to issue a protective order (ie, a restraining order) to the victim. Generally, a protective order is issued when the victim proves, beyond a preponderance of the evidence, that she is in imminent danger as a result of past violent acts or threats of violence by the respondent [25]. In the case of elder abuse, an order of protection may be sought by an abused elder who fears for his or her own physical safety and therefore needs protection from his or her abuser.

State statutes vary, but in general the court may be authorized to compel the abuser to do one or more of the following: (1) refrain from having direct or indirect contact with the individual; (2) refrain from abusing a member in the individual's home; (3) refrain from entering a shared residence, even if title is vested or a lease is in the abuser's name; (4) provide alternative housing for the victim and the victim's family; (5) obtain counseling; and (6) provide the victim with money to pay medical expenses, lost wages, moving expenses, court costs, and attorney's fees [5,10,25]. The order of protection sends a signal to abusers that society denounces abusive behavior. For some abusers, hearing from a judge that mistreatment is intolerable and being threatened with imprisonment is enough to deter the individual from committing abusive acts in the future [9].

To invoke protection under a domestic violence statute, an abuse victim or someone authorized to act on the behalf of the individual must file a petition with a court authorized to issue an order of protection. The victim may have a choice to file a petition in civil or criminal court. For example, under Illinois law, an order of protection is a civil proceeding and is issued in civil court [26]. A civil order of protection may be issued in criminal court if the abuser is prosecuted for a crime arising out of the same incident. In this case, an order of protection is tacked onto the criminal proceeding [26].

After the petition is filed, a hearing is held, usually within 2 weeks. In the interim, a temporary order of protection (ie, an emergency restraining order) may be issued and lasts until the initial court hearing. The issuance of a temporary order of protection is dependent on the immediacy and emergent nature of potential harm to the victim [25].

Orders of protection are generally available to anyone abused by a spouse, former spouse, family member, household member, or former household member. Because some states issue orders of protection only against a spouse or former spouse, such statutes limit protection to elders who are not married to their abusers [5]. Some states further limit protection by requiring the initiation of divorce proceedings before issuance. Most states issue orders of protection to victims who are abused by an individual in a shared residence or against a former household member, thus making a protective order a potentially valuable tool for victims of elder abuse [5].

Violation of a protective order is a crime and can result in the abuser's arrest, contempt of court, and charges for any criminal acts committed [10]. The goal is to discourage the abuser from engaging in a cycle of abuse. Problems arise if an order of protection is violated. The victim must enforce the order of protection and is often reluctant to contact the police or initiate enforcement proceedings [9,10].

Protective orders are not always an adequate solution for victims of elder abuse. Assuming an order of protection is issued against a member of the abused elder's household, the order may protect the individual from violence while simultaneously forcing a primary caretaker to leave. If the victim does not have an adequate network of support, the loss a primary caretaker, abusive or not, may force the individual to refrain from obtaining a protective order or force them into an institutional setting [10].

Legal actions against professionals for failing to report elder abuse

Mandatory reporting laws seek to compel interventions in abusive situations by (1) requiring professionals or anyone with a "reasonable belief" of abuse to report it to specific agencies, (2) providing immunity for those reporting in good faith, and (3) triggering investigative reports and services by adult protective service agencies [9]. The inclusion of professionals, such as licensed health care workers and social workers, in the category of those mandated to report suggests a legislative recognition of their access to elderly individuals. Licensed health care workers and social workers are likely to examine and treat injured older Americans and are presumably qualified to identify symptoms and indications of abuse. Additionally, their status as professionals increases the likelihood that an abused elder will confide in them regarding instances of abuse [27].

Criminal liability

Failure to report elder abuse in compliance with the statutory requirements is often categorized as a criminal offense. Criminal enforcement of these laws, however, is virtually non-existent. Prosecutors are rarely aware of the failure to report. Even if knowledge is present, prosecutors have difficulty bringing charges for elder abuse for a myriad of reasons. Generally, there is a lack of funding for successful prosecution [5]. Elder abuse cases are expensive to prosecute because financial and medical experts are often necessary. Additionally, evidentiary issues bar prosecutions because victims may be unavailable, unwilling, or unable to participate in the process [5].

Civil liability

Because criminal prosecution of professionals who fail to comply with their duty to report has been an ineffective tool in compelling compliance, civil liability may prove to be a more effective vehicle for encouraging professionals to report instances of abuse. Civil enforcement is generally seen through malpractice litigation and licensure sanctions. The primary goal of malpractice suits and professional licensure sanctions is to hold professionals accountable for deviations from the standard of care and to deter noncompliance with such accountability [5].

Legal actions against perpetrators of abuse

Civil liability of abusers

The use of civil lawsuits allows victims of elder abuse to sue perpetrators for resulting injuries. Abuse victims can bring suits in tort depending on the type of abuse suffered [11]. Suits for physical abuse may be brought under common law notions of assault and battery. Victims of emotional abuse may bring a suit based on the intentional infliction of emotional distress and assault. Suits for financial exploitation may be brought under the laws of conversion or fraud [5,6].

The effectiveness of civil lawsuits is limited by the fact that victims of abuse must individually file a suit against their abuser (although a guardian or person acting as an agent under a power of attorney may file a lawsuit on behalf of the abused elder) [6]. Victims of elder abuse are reluctant to report abuse and thus are similarly unlikely to initiate a timely and expensive civil proceeding. Additionally, victims of elder abuse may have insufficient resources to pursue legal action. The use of civil laws alone may be an insufficient remedy to combat elder abuse because civil laws only affect the abuser financially. Forcing a perpetrator to compensate the victims financially may not deter the abuser from pursuing a similar course of action against another individual [6].

Criminal liability of abusers

The remedies afforded by criminal laws are broader than civil sanctions. Criminal laws protect the victim from an abusive relationship and punish the perpetrator for engaging in prohibited conduct [6]. Criminalizing elder abuse sends a clear message to perpetrators that society denounces this type of behavior [5]. Additionally, because criminal laws are enforced by the state, the problems associated with victim-initiated litigation are absent [6].

Abuse, neglect, and financial exploitation of elders have been made specific crimes in many states. Research suggests that older Americans are more susceptible to crime, the effects of which are heightened in comparison to the rest of the population [5]. Most states allow the advanced age of the victim to constitute an aggravating circumstance in sentencing [3]. Even without a statute specifically designating old age as an aggravating circumstance, a judge may exercise discretion and enhance a penalty if the judge remains within the normal sentencing guidelines [3,5].

Financial exploitation of older Americans

Financial abuse and exploitation mirror physical and psychologic abuse in many ways. Financial abuse is difficult to detect because there are rarely any witnesses to the behavior other than the victim and the abuser [6]. It includes actions that convert money and property from their rightful owner and can be conducted by friends or strangers [28]. Unknown perpetrators can financially exploit elderly individuals through fright mail, mail fraud, and fraudulent tele-marketing tactics [6].

Fright mail includes any letter that fictitiously illustrates an alarming political matter. The letters seem to be informative but are misleading and clearly designed to scare recipients into sending money for the purported political purpose. Fright mail sent to older Americans is specifically tailored to their political concerns. For example, an older adult may receive letters from an organization claiming social security is on the verge of collapsing and that money is needed to guard against its destruction. Such claims appeal to the emotional and psychologic fears of the elderly [6]. These organizations have escaped liability under current federal laws because they do not promise to spend the money on a particular purpose [6].

Mail fraud deceives victims into spending money on products or services to win a prize. This includes sweepstakes promotions that claim the recipient is already a winner. Although many individuals quickly dispose of such mailings, many older Americans look through such letters because they frequently have more time. Creative marketing tactics and glitzy packages are more likely to draw the attention of older adults who may be isolated and vulnerable [6].

The federal mail fraud statute (formally known as The White-Collar Crime Penalty Enhancement Act of 2002) addresses such schemes by punishing individuals who use the postal service as a means to obtain money or property through false representations. Punishment may include up to 5 years imprisonment, a fine, or both [6,29]. State legislation addresses mail fraud through consumer protection statutes. Some states enhance penalties if victims are advanced in age [6].

Telemarketing fraud, like mail fraud, entices victims to spend money on products or services to win a prize. The only difference between the two is the manner in which the scheme is conducted; telemarketing fraud targets victims over the phone [6].

Elderly individuals are primary targets for telemarketing fraud because they often remain in the home and are responsive to promises for quick money. Once a victim responds to an instance of telemarketing fraud, they become an easy target for future abuse. Individuals who send money pursuant to a telemarketer's request are placed onto a "mooch" list and contacted repeatedly with similar requests [6].

In 1994, Congress reacted to telemarketing fraud by enacting the Senior Citizens Against Marketing Scams Act (SCAMS), a statute designed to protect elders from fraud and offer restitution to victims [6,30]. SCAMS incorporates provisions of the federal mail fraud act and adds an additional 5 years to any prison sentence if the scheme is conducted through telemarketing. SCAMS further protects older Americans by adding 10 years to a prison sentence if the victim is over the age of 55 [6,30]. SCAMS requires restitution to the victim equivalent to the amount of losses proximately caused by the abuser's conduct [6,30].

States have attacked telemarketing fraud through the use of consumer protection statutes. These statutes differ dramatically in the amount of protection afforded. Some statutes specifically criminalize fraudulent and deceptive telemarketing schemes and allow prosecution for a felony or monetary damages for violation of the statute [6]. Other protections include requirements that telemarketing companies register with the state; monitoring phone calls during certain time periods; requiring companies to offer a refund any time a credit card is used over the telephone; and authorizing the attorney general to issue an injunction to enforce the statute, seek civil money penalties, and restitution [6]. Because the protection offered by each state varies, telemarketing companies can avoid serious penalties by moving their organization across state lines [6].

Summary

Lillian, Glenda, Frank, Jerry and John, the individuals in the examples at the beginning of this article, are representative of older adults in the United States. More must be done to protect them. Older Americans constitute the fastest growing segment of the United States population and may account for 20% of the nation in the year 2050; however, the federal government has taken minimal action to identify and solve their problems. Due to the federal government's inaction, states have become the primary engine for combating elder abuse. This is most often seen through adult protective services, which primarily consist of mandatory reporting laws, involuntary interventions, and educational programs.

Although there are some similarities in state laws, the creation of 52 (ie, all 50 states, the District of Columbia, and Guam) different methods of response to elder abuse results in disparate protection of older Americans across the nation.

Funding is the primary roadblock to the successful execution of state laws targeting domestic elder abuse. Without federal financial assistance, the states are hard pressed to fight domestic elder abuse. If the United States Elder Justice Act of 2003 is passed, it may fill in the gaps left by current federal legislation and may provide a cohesive link between current state statutes by implementing a uniform method of response to domestic elder abuse and by providing adequate funding to the states to rectify instances of abuse.

References

[1] House Select Committee on Aging. Elder abuse: an examination of a hidden problem. 97th Congress, 1st Session; 1981.

[2] House Subcommittee on Health Long-Term Care. Elder abuse: a decade of shame and inaction: a report by the Chairman of the Subcommittee on Health and Long-Term Care of the Select Committee on Aging, House of Representatives, 101st Congress, 2nd Session; 1990.

[3] Adams Jr WE. The intersection of elder law and criminal law: more traffic than one might assume. Stetson Law Rev 2001;30:1331–52.

[4] US Department of Commerce, Bureau of the Census, Statistical Abstract of the United States. 1995 at 15 (Table No. 14, Resident Population, by Age and Sex: 1970 to 1994).

[5] Moskowitz S. Saving granny from the wolf: elder abuse and neglect-the legal framework. Conn Law Rev 1998;31:77–201.

[6] Moore S, Schaefer J. Remembering the forgotten ones: protecting the elderly from financial abuse. San Diego Law Review 2004;41:505–91.

[7] US Department of Commerce, Bureau of the Census, Statistical Abstract of the United States. 2003 at 14 (Table No. 12, Resident Population Projections by Sex and Age: 2005 to 2050).

[8] Teaster PB. A response to the abuse of vulnerable adults: the 2000 survey of state adult protective services. Available at: www.elderabusecenter.org. Accessed September 30, 2004.

[9] Adelman RD, Lachs MS, Breckman R. Elder abuse and neglect. In: Ammerman RT, Hersen M, editors. Assessment of family violence: a clinical and legal sourcebook. 2nd edition. New York: John Wiley & Sons; 1999. p. 271–86.

[10] Senate Special Committee on Aging. An advocate's guide to laws and programs addressing elder abuse: an information paper by the Special Committee on Aging of the United States Senate. 1991.

[11] Moskowitz S. Golden age in the golden state: contemporary legal developments in elder abuse and neglect. Loyola Los Angeles Law Rev 2003;36:589–666.

[12] National Center on Elder Abuse web site. Available at: www.elderabusecenter.org. Accessed September 30, 2004.

[13] Geroff AJ, Olshaker JS. Elder abuse. In: Olshaker JS, Jackson MC, Smock WS, editors. Forensic emergency medicine. Philadelphia: Lippincott Williams & Wilkins; 2001. p. 173–202.

[14] Older Americans Personal Health Education and Training Act, 42 U.S.C. § 3058. 2004.

[15] Title XX of the Social Security Act, 42 U.S.C. § 1397. 2004.

[16] Breaux J, Hatch O. Confronting elder abuse, neglect and exploitation: the need for elder justice legislation. Elder Law J 2003;11:207–71.

[17] Elder Justice Act of 2002, S. 2933, 107th Congress, 2002; Elder Justice Act of 2003, S. 333, H.R. 2490, 108th Congress, 2003.

[18] Administration on Aging web site. Available at: www.aoa.gov/eldfam/Elder_Rights/Elder_Abuse/Elder_Abuse.asp. Accessed September 27, 2004.

[19] Rathbone-McCuan E. Elder abuse within the context of intimate violence. Univ Missouri Kansas City Law Rev 2000;69:215–26.

[20] Garfield AS. Elder abuse and the states' adult protective services response: time for a change in California. Hastings Law J 1991;42:859–937.

[21] Velick MD. Mandatory reporting statutes: a necessary yet underutilized response to elder abuse. Elder Law J 1995;3:165–90.

[22] American Medical Association. AMA policy finder, Council on Ethical and Judicial Affairs, H-515.965. Family and intimate partner violence. Available at: www.ama-assn.org. Accessed November 1, 2004.

[23] American Medical Association. AMA Policy Finder, Code of Medical Ethics, Ethical Opinion E-2.02. Abuse of spouses, children, elderly persons, and others at risk. Available at: www/ama-assn.org. Accessed November 1, 2004.

[24] Andrews M. The elderly in guardianship: a crisis of constitutional proportions. Elder Law J 1997;5:75–115.

[25] Lederman C, Malik N. Family violence: a report on the state of the research. Florida Bar J 1999;73:58–62.

[26] The Illinois Domestic Violence Act of 1986, 750 ILL. COMP. STAT. §§ 60/102–401. 2004.

[27] Brandl B, Meuer T. Domestic abuse in later life. Elder Law J 2000;8:297–322.

[28] Dessin C. Financial abuse of the elderly. Ida Law Rev 2000;36:203–26.

[29] The White-Collar Crime Penalty Enhancement Act of 2002, 18 U.S.C. §§ 1341–2. 2002.

[30] The Senior Citizens Against Marketing SCAMS Act of 1994, 18 U.S.C. §§ 2325–7. 2000.

ELSEVIER
SAUNDERS

Clin Geriatr Med 21 (2005) 399–412

CLINICS IN
GERIATRIC
MEDICINE

Forensic Markers in Elder Female Sexual Abuse Cases

Ann W. Burgess, RN, DNSc, FAAN[a],
Nancy P. Hanrahan, PhD, RN, CS[b],*, Timothy Baker, PhD[c]

[a]William Connell School of Nursing, Boston College, 120 Commonwealth Avenue,
Chestnut Hill, MA 02467, USA
[b]Center for Health Outcomes and Policy Research, University of Pennsylvania School of Nursing,
420 Guardian Drive, NEB #337, Philadelphia, PA 19104, USA
[c]Data Integrity, Inc., 228 Highland Avenue, West Newton, MA 02465, USA

The 2002 National Crime Victimization Survey (NCVS) reported 247,730 victims of rape, attempted rape, or sexual assault in the United States [1]. Although evidence exists that older adults are victims of sexual assault and rape [2–12], the scope of the problem and the prevalence and correlates of these sex crimes are relatively unknown. Although age is a factor in the NCVS database, few cases of persons over 60 years of age are reported, which makes the determination of prevalence problematic [13]. Risk factors for sexual victimization in the older adult age group are often inferred from the younger cohort [14].

Sexual victimization is under-reported in all age groups. Older victims' threshold for reporting sexual victimization is lower than the younger cohort [15–18]. Fear of retaliation and the victim's shame combined with asexual stereotypes of older adults by family, caretakers, clinicians, and police prevent detection and delay reporting [15]. Although these are unique barriers to recording the prevalence of rape in the older adult population, the clinical literature is vague about the substantial impact that physiologic and emotional

This project was supported in part by grant no. 2001-IJ-CX-K015 and grant no. 2003-WG-BX-1007 awarded by the National Institute of Justice, Office of Justice Programs, Department of Justice.

* Corresponding author.

E-mail address: nancyp@nursing.upenn.edu (N.P. Hanrahan).

aging has on gathering adequate evidence to support claims of sexual victimization of older adults [8].

To address the scant attention given to elder victims of sexual abuse, the National Institute for Justice funded a working group project to gather experts from medicine, law enforcement, criminal justice, corrections, forensics, nursing, social work, and psychology to address the lack of information about sexual abuse in the elderly population. The purpose was to describe forensic makers of intentional sexual injuries in the older adult female population. This article summarizes the experts' synthesis of essential concepts necessary for constructing a national database using the following categories: mechanisms and patterns of injury in elder sexual abuse cases, forensic evidence, the characteristics and patterns of behavior of the perpetrators, the characteristics and patterns of behavior observed in the victim, the criminal justice process, and outcomes in elder sexual abuse cases.

Prevalence estimates of rape

The NCVS is a national reference of the state of interpersonal violence and crime statistics, specifically rape and sexual assault. Nine out of 10 rape victims are female [2]. Almost 20 million women and almost 3 million men have reported being a victim of rape sometime in their life [3]. Although most rape victims are female and white (82.5%), blacks are 10% more likely to be attacked and raped than whites [1]. There are many common factors among the various age cohorts, but little empiric evidence exists to establish reliable and valid prevalence rates of rape and sexual assault for older adults.

According to the NCVS, only 39% of rapes and sexual assaults are reported to law enforcement officials, and only 6% of rapists are convicted [1]. Victims report they are silent because of the shame and humiliation of public exposure and the fear of reprisal from an assailant [1,5]. "Hidden rape" is especially relevant to the experience of older women [4]. Pavlik et al [6] explored a database owned by the Texas Department of Protective and Regulatory Services. There were 43,250 older adults reporting 62,000 allegations of adult mistreatment and neglect. The study measured the distribution of abuse types reported and population prevalence estimates of each abuse type by age and sex. Sexual abuse accounted for 0.01% ($n = 584$). Acierno et al [7] conducted a retrospective study using National Women's Study (NWS) survey data to compare assault characteristics of 549 women 55 to 89 years of age with 2669 women 18 to 35 years of age [7]. The researchers reported a higher prevalence rate of rape in the younger cohort (17.4%) versus in the older women (6.2%). Victimization prevalence rates have a high degree of bias due to differences in the way older women report or perceive rape as compared with younger women [6,7].

Older victims' threshold for reporting sexual victimization is lower than the younger cohort [7–10]. Due to more restrictive cultural views of the sexuality, older victims do not report sex crimes and are more likely to self-blame and feel humiliation than younger victims [11]. Sexual stereotypes (eg, viewing older adults as asexual or not sexually attractive) of older adults by family, caretakers, clinicians, police, and others prevent detection and result in delayed reporting. These are unique barriers to recording the prevalence of rape in the older adult population [12,13]. Victims of rape share devastating short- and long-term physical and emotional effects from the trauma. Post-traumatic stress disorder (PTSD), depression, and physical problems are common to all age groups [5,14,15].

Select studies of sexually victimized older adults

Twenty cases of referred nursing home resident victims of sexual assault were analyzed by Burgess et al [16]. Eleven of 20 victims died within 12 months of the assault, suggesting that nursing home victims of sexual abuse are often physically and emotionally fragile and have severe traumatic reactions to assault. A similar conclusion was found by other researchers [17–21].

Using data from the NCVS for 1992 through 1994, Bachman et al [21] examined robbery and assault against older Americans. They intended to define differential patterns of risk by contextual characteristics of the victimization, including place of occurrence, weapon presence, injuries sustained, medical care required, and victim's relationship to the offender. They found that when compared with younger women, older women are more likely to sustain injuries as a result of a violent attack and are more likely to require medical care for these injuries. They found that older women are more likely to be assaulted in their homes than in any other location by intimates and other family members.

Teaster [10] surveyed administrators in all 50 states in the United States regarding the abuse and neglect of older adults. There were a total of 472,813 reports of abuse or neglect, which included self-neglect (39%), caregiver neglect (19%), financial abuse (13%), physical abuse (11%), emotional abuse (7%), and sexual abuse (1%). Most (56%) were women; 65% were white, 17% were black, and 10.5% were Hispanic. Adults 80 years of age and older (46.5%) suffered the greatest share of abuse, with 60.7% of reports from domestic settings. The perpetrator was usually male (52%), with the age distribution as follows: 36 to 50 years of age, 24.8%; 36 to 50 years of age, 24.8%; 18 to 35 years of age, 18.5%; and <18 years of age, 5.9%. In 62% of the cases, the perpetrator was related to the victim; of these, 30.2% were intimate/spouse partners, and 17.6% were adult children.

Muram [18] compared 53 women 55 years of age or older with 53 women aged 18 to 45. Both groups were victims of rape. In 28% of older women, injuries sustained to the genital area were severe enough to warrant surgical repair. The link between sexual violence, the deterioration of mental and physical health, and the subsequent higher need for health care is not empirically established for older adults. However, a sexual assault history has been shown to increase the need for and use of health care services.

Stein and Barret-Connor [22] examined the association of a prior sexual assault history with physical illness in older age. The sample was from 1359 community-dwelling men ($n = 533$) and women ($n = 829$), with an average age of 74 years. Using a self-administered sexual assault questionnaire during a clinic visit, the researchers asked, "In your lifetime, has anyone ever tried to pressure or force you to have unwanted sexual contact?" If the respondent admitted to being assaulted, they were asked if repeated sexual assaults had occurred and if they had received counseling. Sexual assault rates for women were 12.7%, with 21.9% of these women reporting repeated experiences. Only 3.8% of the women reported receiving counseling. Women who had histories of sexual abuse had a significant higher risk for arthritis, breast cancer, and thyroid disease [22].

Methods

The study was a retrospective analysis of 125 cases of elder sexual abuse. Experts were invited to join a working group to determine essential forensic markers (FMs) unique to older adult victims of sexual abuse. To participate, experts were required to (1) have direct clinical, administrative, investigative, or legal experience with older adult sexual victims; (2) submit at least five substantiated elder sexual abuse cases for analysis before a scheduled working group meeting; and (3) bring two nonprosecuted or unfounded cases for discussion at the working group meeting.

The following is a summary of all the experts that attended the working group meeting: eight attorneys, seven Sexual Assault Nurse Examiners, three investigators (police, detective, FBI), three administrators (Adult Protective Services), six clinicians (social worker, physician, nurse practitioner, and nurses), three older adult consumers and advocates. The experts represented the following regions of the United States: New England, Middle Atlantic, West North Central Division, West South Central Division, East North Central Division, South Atlantic Division, and Pacific Division. Cases submitted by the experts had a similar geographic distribution.

Before the meeting, the experts used the Comprehensive Sexual Assault Assessment Tool (CSAAT) [23] to record data on their cases. Data sources included clinical reports from sexual assault forensic examiners, investigative reports, photographs or colposcopy slides, and reports from law enforcement or the prosecutor's office on the outcome of the case. Names were redacted, and a coded number was given to each case. Internal Review Board approval was secured from Boston College Institution Review Board.

Univariate statistics, Pearson correlations, and chi square analysis were used to examine significant relationships. SPSS software was used for the analysis. During the group meeting, summary statistics of the 125 submitted cases were interpreted by the experts. The results of the analysis of the 125 female cases of elder sexual abuse are presented below with the caveat that these preliminary data have limitations. The instrument used to collect the data (the CSAAT) was not specifically designed for use with elderly sexual assault victims, the sample was not nationally representative, the case files were derived from various sources, and a convenience sampling method was used.

Results

Victim characteristics and patterns of behavior

The mean age of the 125 women studied was 78.5 years (Table 1). The majority was Caucasian (83%); 12% were African American, 3% were Hispanic, and 2% were Asian. Sixty-six percent were widowed, 17% were single, 10% were married, and 5% were divorced. Most (93.9%) spoke English as a primary language.

The elderly women were generally small in stature and weight and suffered from a physical or mental disability (49%). Forty-three percent of the women lived alone at the time of the incident, 38% lived in nursing homes, and 6% were in assisted living situations. The remainder lived with a spouse or family member (10%) or in some other place (3%).

Mechanisms of injury

The offender used his/her hand as the primary mechanism of physical injury to the nongenital area of the victim's body in this sample (Table 2). Blunt, force

Table 1
Demographic characteristics of elder victims of sexual assault

	N	n (%)
Race	118	
Asian		2 (1.7)
Black		14 (11.9)
Caucasian		98 (83.1)
Hispanic		4 (3.4)
Marital status	85	
Single		14
Married		9
Divorced		5
Widowed		57
Victim has a physical disability	105	56 (48.7)
Victim has a mental disability	115	52 (45.2)
Victim resides	121	
Alone		51 (42.5)
With spouse/family		11 (9.1)
Nursing home		46 (38)
Assisted living		7 (5.8)
Other		4 (3.3)

Mean age, 78.48 years; mode, 78; median, 78; min, 60; max, 98.

Table 2
Mechanisms of injury

	N^a	n (%)
Con subterfuge or ploy	90	21 (23.3)
Blitz (no warning)	97	72 (74.2)
Mere presence	91	65 (71.4)
Weapon	94	17 (18.1)
Threat	87	36 (41.4)
Medications	93	3 (3.2)
Bound victim	77	8 (10.4)
Gagged victim	81	11 (13.6)
Blindfolded victim	81	8 (9.8)
Abducted victim	81	11 (13.6)
Bribery	98	3 (3.1)
Psychologic coercion	97	18 (18.6)
Victim clothing removed	89	70 (78.7)
Offender took off victim's clothes	68	57 (93.8)
Offender used alcohol or drugs	68	31 (45.6)
Offender forced victim to use alcohol	87	4 (4.6)

[a] Not all cases recorded the items.

trauma was used to grab, push, punch, restrain, or slap the victim. Thumb or finger marks were noted on forensic examination. Injury to the genital area was caused by the offender's hand, fingers, mouth, or penis. In approximately 12% of victims, the perpetrator used a foreign object (such as a shower head).

Offenders reportedly brought weapons (eg, a knife or a gun) in 17% of cases and disabled a telephone in about 16% of the cases. Bindings were brought to the scene in about 10% of the cases, and gloves were used in about 7% of the cases. In one nursing home case, a coat hanger was used to intimidate, beat, and penetrate the victim.

Patterns of injury

Elderly victims suffered a significant amount of injury to nongenital parts of their body (Table 3). Over half had at least one part of their body indicating bruising or abrasion (52%). Thirty-eight percent of the victims had injury to their head, and the arms were injured in 31% of cases. Other target areas were the legs (24%), the chest (22%), abdomen (13%), and other (20%).

Nearly half of the cases had vaginal trauma (46%), with about one third of the cases indicating bruising to the labia minora, posterior fourchette, and labia majora. Trauma was noted to one genital area 12% of the time, to two genital areas 12% of the time, to three genital areas 15% of the time, and to four to seven genital areas 19% of the time.

Various sexual acts were forced on the victims. Women reported being kissed (17%), having their breasts fondled (32%), being orally penetrated (13%), being vaginally penetrated (78%), and being anally penetrated (24%).

Table 3
Patterns of genital and physical trauma

	N	n (%)
Genital trauma		
Labia majora	90	28 (31.1)
Labia minora	90	34 (37.8)
Clitoris	85	4 (4.7)
Posterior fourchette	86	32 (37.2)
Fossa nauvicularis	84	16 (19)
Periurethral	83	9 (10.8)
Vestibule	81	8 (9.9)
Vagina	91	42 (46.2)
Hymen	84	7 (8.3)
Cervix	81	10 (12.3)
Perineum	85	11 (12.9)
Anus	90	15 (16.7)
Rectum	83	7 (8.4)
Physical trauma		
Head	114	43 (37.7)
Arms	110	34 (30.9)
Chest	110	24 (21.8)
Abdomen	106	14 (13.2)
Legs	107	26 (24.3)
Other	83	17 (20.5)

Forensic examination

There were only 46 cases in the study with forensic data available. Of the 46 cases, 16 (35%) had positive evidence for the presence of sperm in the vagina (13/45), on anal swab (5/45), or on oral swab (1/44).

Similar to younger rape victims, elderly victims had a wide response to the rape examination. During the forensic examination, 35% of the victims were noted to be trembling, 26% were noted as quiet or tense, 17% gave brief responses, and 4% were noted as reluctant. Concerning expressive demeanor, 36% were noted as responsive, and 35% were tearful or sobbing. Twenty-one percent were agitated, and 7% were angry.

Elderly victims were not routinely assessed for the psychologic impact of the sexual assault. A psychologic assessment for symptoms of PTSD was completed in fewer than 23% of the cases.

Offender characteristics and patterns of behavior

Although most of the offenders were male (93%), there were some female perpetrators (7%) (Table 4). Over half of the offenders were Caucasian (51%), 40% were African American, 6% were Hispanic, and 2% were other. Offenders ranged in age from 15 to 85 years, with a mean age of 37 years. Few had physical disabilities (5%) or mental disabilities (14%). In 31% of the cases, the offender was reported as having a sexual dysfunction. The offender was reported to

Table 4
Offender characteristics and patterns of behavior

	Mean	Median	Range
Offender age, yr	37.24	31	15–85
Offender weight, lb	171.57	167	
Offender height, in	68.40	68.3	

	N	n (%)
Male gender	105	97 (92.4)
Race/ethnicity		
White	93	47 (50.5)
Black	93	38 (40.9)
Hispanic	93	6 (6.5)
Other	93	2 (2.2)
Unique features	66	15 (22.7)
Physical disability	87	5 (5.7)
Mental disability	86	13 (15.1)
Relationship to victim		
Victim known	108	63 (58.3)
Caretaker	62	16 (25.8)
Resident of nursing home	62	13 (21)
Stranger	62	2 (3.2)

be on alcohol or drugs in close to half of the cases (44%). There were multiple offenders in about 9% of the offenses, and 44% of the offenders had multiple offenses.

In 59% of the cases, the relationship between offender and victim was known. Almost half of the offenders were acquaintances (48%), 26% were caretakers, 19% were residents in the same nursing home, and only 3% were strangers. Robbery was present in over 34% of the cases; items of value were taken 34% of the time, and personal items were taken 25% of the time. Control of the victim was managed by the mere presence of the offender in 72% of the cases. Beating or battery occurred in 45% of the cases, with threats used in 40%, a weapon in 19%, and psychologic coercion in 18%. The victim was controlled by being gagged (13%), bound (10%), blindfolded (9%), medicated (3%), bribed (3%), or abducted (2%).

Criminal justice process and outcomes

Based on 120 of 125 cases in which there were adequate data for coding, the reporting and disposition of these offenses went as follows (Table 5). Law enforcement was notified in 96% of the cases. There were 88 out of 117 offenders (75%) identified, 65 out of 116 (56%) arrested, and 64 out of 116 (55%) charged. Half of these cases (57 of 113 with data) were prosecuted.

Table 5
Criminal justice process and outcomes

	N	n (%)
Police notified	120	116 (96.7)
Offender identified	117	88 (75.2)
Offender arrested	116	65 (56)
Offender charged	116	64 (55.2)
Offender tried	113	54 (50.4)
Plea bargain	96	33 (34.4)
Guilty	113	26 (23)
Sexual offense charged	71	19 (26.8)
Lesser sexual charge	71	19 (26.8)
Rape charged	71	33 (46.5)
Murder charge	68	15 (22.1)
Other charges	68	32 (42.9)

Of the 113 cases, about one out of four was found guilty. A plea bargain was reached in 32 of the 113 cases (28%), and 55 of the 113 (48%) did not have charges filed or were found not guilty. In reviewing 71 of the cases with criminal charges listed, 33 (46%) were charged with rape, 19 (26%) were charged with a lesser sexual charge, and 19 (26%) were charged with a crime other than sexual assault. Other charges in addition or in lieu of a sexual abuse charge included 15 cases that carried a murder charge, 27 that carried a burglary/robbery charge, three that carried a kidnapping charge, and two that carried a battery charge.

Forensic markers significant in the prosecution of cases

Correlation analyses were performed on the 125 cases of sexually abused women to compare offenders who were charged and found guilty and those who were not. The younger the victim was, the greater was the likelihood that the offender would be found guilty. If the victim were tearful or sobbing during the forensic examination, if a urinary tract infection was present, and if a psychologic assessment for PTSD was completed, there was a greater likelihood of an offender being found guilty. If the victim had a mental disability (particularly dementia), there was a lower likelihood that the offender would be charged and found guilty.

If evidence were destroyed, there was a lower likelihood that the offender would be charged and found guilty. This was particularly true if the victim urinated, defecated, changed clothes, or brushed her teeth. If the victim took a bath or shower, there was less likelihood of being charged ($r = -0.22$, $P = 0.042$) and found guilty ($r = -0.20$, $P = 0.064$). With forensic evidence being destroyed, there was a correlation of -0.26 ($P = 0.011$) with being charged and correlation of -0.24 ($P = 0.073$) with being found guilty.

If sperm were present, there was a greater likelihood of the offender being charged and found guilty. Offenders of victims with trauma to the body had a greater likelihood of being charged and found guilty. This was particularly true with trauma to the head, the abdomen, the chest, and the legs. The greater the number of body parts where trauma was noted, the greater was the likelihood of charges being brought and the person being found guilty.

The victim's living situation had an impact on the outcome in the criminal justice system. If the victim lived in an assisted living situation, there was a lower likelihood that charges would be brought and the person found guilty. If the victim lived alone, the opposite was true. If the victim lived in a nursing home, there was a lesser likelihood that the person would be charged ($r = -0.19$, $P = 0.035$) or be found guilty ($r = -0.17$, $P = 0.070$).

If the offender was tall, of a different race from the victim, and used alcohol or drugs, there was a greater likelihood of the offender being charged and found guilty. If the offender controlled the victim by battery and beatings, there was a greater likelihood of being charged and found guilty. The amount of force was significantly related to being charged and found guilty.

Comparison of community-based victims and nursing home victims

Over one third of the cases (38%) involved nursing home residents. Nursing home victims were significantly older than the rest of the sample. Most of the nursing home victims were Caucasian and widowed, and just over half of the perpetrators were the same race as the victims. The overwhelming majority of nursing home victims had a physical and mental disability when compared with non-nursing home victims. Most of the nursing home victims were assaulted in their bed. Correlations comparing the 46 nursing home cases with the 79 non-nursing home cases revealed the following: (1) Nursing home victims were more likely to have their breasts fondled, be more agitated, be raped by a male nursing home resident, be victimized by an offender with mental disabilities, have items of value stolen, and be controlled by the offender's mere presence. (2) Nursing home victims were less likely to have a rape kit used for evidence collection, to have sperm found, have less physical trauma, be tested for sexually transmitted diseases, be controlled by physical force of the offender, and have resident-offender charged with an offense or be found guilty. (3) Potential evidence was often found to have been destroyed in nursing home victims (eg, being bathed before a forensic examination, sheets sent to the laundry, and so forth); nursing home victims were less likely to have been examined with a colposcope or have an evidence kit collected.

The average age of perpetrators in nursing homes was significantly higher than the total sample because some of the perpetrators were nursing home residents. When they were removed from the population, there was no significant difference in perpetrator age between the two samples. None of the nursing home resident perpetrators were charged with any offense.

Discussion

Nearly 80% of the elder victims in our study lived alone or in nursing homes. The nursing home residents were older and more likely than the non-nursing home residents to be physically and mentally disabled. This combined with the fact that the perpetrator was more likely to be known to the victim as an acquaintance, family member, or staff emphasizes the higher level of vulnerability in this age group and the need to legislate protective laws such as criminal background checks for potential employees of nursing homes or residential services and to support elder protective services. Frail elders are more vulnerable to abuse and to sexual predators. In this study, the offender dominated the elder victims by mere presence, and force was used in nearly half of the cases. If the victim resisted, the perpetrator increased the force. Nearly half of the offenders in our study used alcohol or drugs and had a history of previous assaults.

How does our FM study compare with two national surveys of violence against women (Table 6)? The NWS is a longitudinal survey with a probability sample of 4009 American women of which 549 were 55 years of age or older. The purpose of the NWS was to identify risk factors for rape, physical assault,

Table 6
Comparison of studies of older women sexually victimized

	Forensic Markers Study[a] (n = 125)	NCVS[b] 1992–2002 rape victims > 60 years old (n = 8642)	The National Women's Study[c] (n = 549)
Victims			
Mean/SD age	78.4	72.2	67
Female, %	100	74.6	100
Caucasians, %	83.1	73.0	83
Black, %	11.9	12.3	8.5
Setting			
Domestic, %	42.5	40	ND
Institutional, %	38	ND	ND
Other, %	19.5	ND	ND
Perpetrators (% male)	92.4	100	ND
Forced vaginal rape	78	ND	5.3
Forced oral rape	13.4	ND	.5
Forced anal rape	23.9	ND	.2
Forced digital rape	11.6	ND	2.2
Physical assault with weapon	15.7	0	3.5
Physical assault w/o a weapon	84.3	100	2.6
Perpetrator known to the victim	58.3	52.3	9.1
Rape reported to authorities	96.7	44	9.1
Charges made	55.2	50	ND

[a] Forensic Marker Study based on contributed cases by experts.
[b] National Crime Victimization Study (NCVS) is a weighted sample from 1992–2002 of women 60 years and older who were sexually abused or assaulted.
[c] The National Women's Study is a subgroup of 549 women over 55 from the larger sample of 4009.

and PTSD [15]. The NCVS data from 1992 through 2002 was used to study female sexual assault victims over 55 years of age (n = 8642, weighted) using the National Archive of Criminal Justice online access forum [1]. The NCVS is the most commonly referenced database on the prevalence of rates and types of violent crime in the United States [1]. The FM study (n = 125) had an older sample and higher percentages in terms of recorded intentional injury, forced sex acts, use of weapons, perpetrator known to victim, rape reported to authority, and prosecution success. Although the average age of subjects in the FM was slightly older than in the other studies, the basic demographic information is comparable with the NWS and NCVS. The most important observation is the lack of detailed data available at the national level on the sexual victimization of elders. Although these differences may be due to sampling bias in our study or to the undersampling of the NCVS and NWS, there is a need to expand the national database to include details of forced intentional sexual injury of elders.

Forensic evidence was lacking in our study for several reasons: (1) Some jurisdictions did not process rape kits because a suspect was not identified, (2) standard protocol for the collection of forensic evidence was destroyed, and (3) state-of-the-art forensic equipment was not used in the forensic examination. In many cases, no pharyngeal or anal tests were performed, vaginal tests were performed in only about one in four victims, and testing for STDs was rarely performed.

Health care providers constitute the front line for identification and intervention when an elderly victim needs assessment for sexual abuse. Policy for standards of care is critical. There are various forensic examination models available (eg, the Sexual Assault Nurse Examiner or sexual response teams). Systematic documentation of the evidence provides a credible record for enduring the demands of the court process. Further study is warranted on the risk factors and impact of sexual abuse of male and female elderly persons and on the motivational intent of the sex offender.

The Sexual Assault Nurse Examiner (SANE) training program provides a national standard for evaluating and documenting forensic evidence related to sex crimes [24,25]. The SANE procedures systematically document the evidence that has a good record for enduring the demands of the court process [26]. Victims in our study did not have evidence collected or processed adequately, often because of the delays in detecting or report of the crime. Using the SANE procedure would promote a standard of practice once the sexual crime was identified and would improve the prosecution of these crimes.

Summary

Understanding how intentional sexual injuries are inflicted on older adults is a growing concern as the population over 65 increases. This study contributes critical information to guide the identification of physical and psychologic markers of elder sexual abuse to be integrated by law enforcement as forensic medical evidence. Findings from this study will be used to educate health care professions about elder sexual abuse, which we hope will promote early detection. Policy implications for monitoring and protecting elders needs to include criminal background checks on staff caring for elders in nursing homes or performing services in the homes of elders. Building knowledge about the unique psychologic and physical characteristics of sexually traumatized elders, outcomes (particularly exacerbation of comorbid conditions and death), and the effectiveness of interventions is essential for future research and policy development.

References

[1] Rennison CM, Rand MR. Criminal victimization, 2002. Washington, DC: United States Department of Justice Office of Justice Programs; 2003.

[2] RAINN. Rape, abuse & incest national network statistics. Washington, DC: Rape, Abuse & Incest National Network; 2003.

[3] Tjaden P, Thoennes N. Full report of the prevalence, incidence, and consequence of violence against women. Washington, DC: United States Department of Justice and the Center for Disease Control and Prevention; 2000.

[4] Falk B, Hasselt VB, Hersen M. Assessment of posttraumatic stress disorder in older victims of rape. J Clin Geropsychol 1997;3:157–71.

[5] Kilpatrick DG, Acierno R. Mental health needs of crime victims: epidemiology and outcomes. J Trauma Stress 2003;16:119–32.

[6] Pavlik VN, Hyman DJ, Festa NA, et al. Quantifying the problem of abuse and neglect in adults: analysis of a statewide database. J Am Geriatr Soc 2001;49:45–8.

[7] Acierno R, Gray M, Best C, et al. Rape and physical violence: comparison of assault characteristics in older and younger adults in the National Women's Study. J Trauma Stress 2001;14:685–95.

[8] Burgess AW, Prentky RA, Dowdell EB. Sexual predators in nursing homes. J Psychosoc Nurs Ment Health Serv 2000;38:26–35.

[9] Norris FH. Epidemiology of trauma: frequency and impact of different potentially traumatic events on different demographic groups. J Consult Clin Psychol 1992;60:409–18.

[10] Teaster PB. A response the abuse of vulnerable adults: The 2000 Survey of State Adult Protective Services. Washington, DC: National Center on Elder Abuse; 2000.

[11] Benbow SM, Haddad PM. Sexual abuse of the elderly mentally ill. Postgrad Med J 1993;69: 803–7.

[12] Koss MP, Graham JR, Kirkhart K, et al. Outcome of eclectic psychotherapy in private psychological practice. Am J Psychother 1983;37:400–10.

[13] Koss MP, Bachar KJ, Hopkins CQ. Restorative justice for sexual violence: repairing victims, building community, and holding offenders accountable. Ann N Y Acad Sci 2003;989:384–96 [discussion 441–5].

[14] Gray MJ, Acierno R. Symptom presentation of older adult crime victims: description of a clinical sample. J Anxiety Disord 2002;16:299–309.

[15] Acierno R, Resnick H, Kilpatrick DG, et al. Risk factors for rape, physical assault, and posttraumatic stress disorder in women: examination of differential multivariate relationships. J Anxiety Disord 1999;13:541–63.

[16] Burgess AW, Dowdell EB, Prentky R, et al. Sexual abuse of nursing home residents. Journal of Psychosocial Nursing Mental Health Service 2000;38(6):10–8.

[17] Cartwright PS. Reported sexual assault in Nashville-Davidson County, Tennessee, 1980–1982. Am J Obstet Gynecol 1986;154:1064–8.

[18] Muram D, Miller K, Cutler A. Sexual assault of the elderly victim. J Interpersonal Violence 1992;7:70–6.

[19] Cartwright PS. Factors that correlate with injury sustained by survivors of sexual assault. Obstet Gynecol 1987;70:44–6.

[20] Cartwright PS, Moore RA. The elderly victim of rape. South Med J 1989;82:988–9.

[21] Bachman R, Dillaway H, Lachs MS. Violence against the elderly. Res Aging 1998;20:183–99.

[22] Stein MB, Barrett-Connor E. Sexual assault and physical health: findings from a population-based study of older adults. Psychosom Med 2000;62:838–43.

[23] Burgess AW, Fawcett J. The comprehensive sexual assault assessment tool. Nurse Practitioner 1996;21:66, 71–6, 78.

[24] Stermac LE, Stirpe TS. Efficacy of a 2-year-old sexual assault nurse examiner program in a Canadian hospital. J Emerg Nurs 2002;28:18–23.

[25] Du Mont J, Parnis D. Forensic nursing in the context of sexual assault: comparing the opinions and practices of nurse examiners and nurses. Appl Nurs Res 2003;16:173–83.

[26] Ledray LE, Arndt S. Examining the sexual assault victim: a new model for nursing care. J Psychosoc Nurs Ment Health Serv 1994;32:7–12.

ELSEVIER
SAUNDERS

CLINICS IN
GERIATRIC
MEDICINE

Clin Geriatr Med 21 (2005) 413–427

Core Data Elements Tracking Elder Sexual Abuse

Nancy P. Hanrahan, RN, PhD[a,*],
Ann W. Burgess, RN, DNSc[b],
Angela M. Gerolamo, RN, MSN[a]

[a]*The Center for Health Outcomes and Policy Research,
University of Pennsylvania School of Nursing, Nursing Education Building, Room 337,
420 Guardian Drive, Philadelphia, PA 19104, USA*
[b]*W.F. Connell School of Nursing, Boston College, 140 Commonwealth Ave.,
Chestnut Hill, MA 02467, USA*

Sexual abuse is a well-established major social and health problem with significant physical and psychologic consequences for its victims. However, large gaps exist in our knowledge about elder sexual abuse. Essential to defining a social problem and tracking the effectiveness of policy interventions is a consistent and valid database. Over the past three decades, a national source of data on incidences of sexual abuse against women and children helped to improve problem recognition and the development of successful programs of prevention and treatment [1]. A first step to identifying and tracking the problem of elder sexual abuse is the development of a database that includes core data elements that are informed by a conceptual framework. The database becomes a relevant laboratory of statistical data that can be continuously refined and serve as a model for informed social planning.

Older adults are victims of sexual abuse, but little is known about the scope of the problem. The identification and prosecution of sexual abuse in the older adult population is confounded by cognitive changes that interfere with communication or physical evidence that mimics the changes of aging. The

This project was supported, in part, by grant no. 2001-IJ-CX-K015 and grant no. 2003-W6-BX-1007 awarded by the National Institute of Justice, Office of Justice Programs, Department of Justice.

* Corresponding author.

E-mail address: nancyp@nursing.upenn.edu (N.P. Hanrahan).

reasons for our failure to tackle forthrightly the problem of elder sexual abuse remain unclear. The obscurity of elder sexual abuse makes it imperative that a database exists to track these crimes against vulnerable elders, particularly those with physical or mental disabilities.

This article describes a research project that used a nominal group method to develop a conceptual framework and core data elements for a database of incidences of elder sexual abuse. The database establishes a standard for detection, assessment, and prosecution of the crime and builds a base from which policy makers can plan and evaluate interventions. The aim of the project was twofold: (1) to identify mechanisms and patterns of injury of elder sexual abuse and (2) through expert consensus, to establish a conceptual foundation from which core data elements are defined as relevant to a database of sexual victimization of elders.

Background

According to the 2001 United States Office of Justice crime report originating from national databases, the high profile of sexual assault and rape in the legal and public health arenas has had a significant positive effect on the identification and prosecution of these crimes. There has been a 30% decrease in sexual victimization crimes nationally [2]. Although elder sexual abuse has been discussed in the clinical literature, there are numerous problems in determining accurate prevalence estimates [3,4]. Symptoms are often under-reported by the victims or under recognized by clinicians [5]. The National Citizens' Coalition for Nursing Home Reform counted 1749 cases over a 3-year period of such abuse in nursing home residents. Furthermore, in 2000, a survey of state adult protective services (APS) by the National Center on Elder Abuse discovered 4150 cases of elder sexual abuse reported by APS administrators [4].

Older adult victims are reluctant to report emotional or psychologic difficulties in general and particularly if they are concerned about credibility or shame associated with sexual assault [6–8]. Moreover, clinicians under-recognize and underdiagnose sexual victimization of older adults [5,7]. Physical manifestations or post-trauma response of sexual abuse are ascribed to normal frailties and maladies of old age or are difficult to diagnose because of medical problems common to aging [5]. Despite growing attention to elder neglect and abuse, empiric research of sexual victimization of older adults is limited [9]. One of the earliest studies of domestic elder sexual abuse by Ramsey-Klawsnik [3] examined 28 women sexually assaulted by those providing care for them. These cases were from APS in Massachusetts. Three quarters of the victims were frail and had physical or mental limitations. Subsequent studies examining domestic [9,10] and nursing home victims of sexual abuse [9,11] found a similar pattern of a frail man or woman with significant mental or physical disability. In a preliminary report of a 5-year study of elder sexual abuse by Teaster et al [9], most of the nursing home cases were not prosecuted because the victim did not have the capacity to participate in the prosecution or substantiate the evidence.

Study method

Clinical, legal, investigative and administrative experts who have experience working with elder victims of sexual abuse gathered in 2002. These experts represented major stakeholders in the identification, assessment, treatment, and legal processing of elder sexual abuse crimes. Before the meeting, each expert was required to submit cases of elder sexual abuse that they examined, supervised, investigated, or prosecuted.

Using a convenience sampling method, 125 cases of female elder sexual abuse victims, 60 years of age and older, were submitted by the experts. The data were collected using the Comprehensive Sexual Assault Assessment Tool (CSAAT). The researchers were aware that the CSAAT instrument lacked specificity for the cohort being studied, and the data were not collected using a single source of data. The sources of the data varied (expert recall, clinical records, court records, prosecutor records, and so forth), as did the person filling out the CSAAT. Given the dearth of existing information about elder sexual abuse, sampling options were restricted. To counterbalance this sampling and data collection limitation, we carefully selected experts with direct clinical, administrative, investigative, or prosecutorial experience. There were eight attorneys, seven Sexual Assault Nurse Examiners (SANE), three investigators (police, detective, FBI), three administrators (APS), six clinicians (social worker, physician, nurse practitioner, and nurses), and three older adult consumers advocates. The experts and the cases submitted represented the following regions of the United States: New England, Middle Atlantic, West North Central Division, West South Central Division, East North Central Division, South Atlantic Division, and Pacific Division.

The original CSAAT was developed to provide a comprehensive and standardized method of documenting rape and sexual assault of women. The four domains included in the instrument are (1) victim data, (2) offender data, (3) investigative data, and (4) case disposition data. An expert panel determined content validity for the CSAAT; however, no psychometric properties are available [12]. The tool is used widely as an instrument for collecting clinical and forensic data when investigating sexual assault crimes. Additionally, the instrument is used to train sexual assault nurse examiners and other health and investigator professionals.

The CSAAT was used by the experts in our project to collect data on cases of elder sexual abuse. The CSAAT provided a base from which to build an instrument that would address unique physical and mental characteristics of the older adult victims, perpetrators, and issues with processing the case through the legal system. We accounted for missing data by using the exact number of cases associated with each variable (see article by Burgess et al, elsewhere in this issue). A few questions were added to the original CSAAT for data collection that were tailored to the older victim's physical and mental status and living situation. For instance, we added questions that assessed for the presence of cognitive and physical disabilities. At a 2-day meeting of the experts, a descriptive summary of the 125 cases was reviewed by the experts and became the stimulus for discussion about the unique characteristics of sexually victimized older adults. The discussion became the groundwork for the conceptual framework and core elements for a database.

After the meeting, the CSAAT was revised and mailed to experts for content validity. The content validity expert panel included four registered nurses trained as SANE; two criminal investigators from the state police and FBI older adult crime profiling units; three attorneys from sex crime units in California, New York, and Massachusetts; a geriatric researcher; a clinical social worker; and a geriatric physician and nurse practitioner. The expert panel was given a working definition of the CSAAT items and was asked to rate the relevance of each item and to note each item as "not relevant," "relevant," or "highly relevant." Reviewers were asked to (1) comment on the wording, vocabulary, sentence structure, and formatting of the item; (2) evaluate the clarity and conciseness of the items and suggest alternative wording; and (3) evaluate the capacity of the instrument to tap vital information about the victim, the offender, the crime, and the disposition of the case. Content revisions accrued until there was 100% agreement that all items were relevant or highly relevant. The final product was named the Comprehensive Sexual Assault Assessment Tool-Elder (CSAAT-E).

Conceptual framework

The conceptual framework explains the pre- and post-assault association between the victim, offender, and assault factors (Fig. 1). Core elements are subsumed under the following domains: (1) victim, (2) offender, (3) crime information, and (4) case disposition. Defining risk factors depends on an accurate assessment of temporal and contextual dimensions to provide safe environments and prevent these crimes. Major changes to the original CSAAT focused on (1) temporality, (2) older adults' physical and mental status, (3) severity of injury, (4) setting of the crime, and (5) documentation of outcomes associated with the assault. Factoring in the temporal dimension of pre- and post-assault is perhaps the most significant revision of the CSAAT. For instance, the time of the examination relative to disclosure and police involvement and outcomes of the event were identified as important components to incorporate into the revised CSAAT.

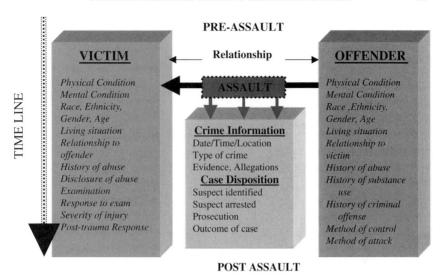

Fig. 1. A conceptual framework of elder vulnerability associated with sexual abuse.

The original instrument did not account for pre-assault and post-assault biopsychosocial characteristics of the victim, which did not allow for the victims' physical, psychologic, and cognitive functioning before the crime to be compared with their functioning after the crime. The temporal dimension establishes a baseline pattern that can be compared with the post-assault phase. Many older adult victims are physically or mentally impaired before the assault, which makes it difficult to causally relate physical or mental injuries after the assault. These patterns are essential data for documenting changes in functional patterns or the emergence of physical or mental symptoms that are potential consequences of the crime.

Another aspect of the temporal dimension is the sequencing of events from assault to disclosure, including information about the time lapse from the incident to a physical examination where forensic evidence is collected. Clarity about who performed the interview and filled out the data collection instrument and the time lapse from victimization to interview and examination is necessary for adequate evidence and prosecution of the case. In many cases of elder sexual abuse, there is long time lapse between the assault, disclosure of the assault, and the collection of forensic evidence. The time lapse may be due to impaired expressive or receptive communication of the victim that delays the recognition of the crime by providers. Providers may not recognize the physical or mental injuries as a consequence of a sexual assault. Delays in recognizing sexual assault may place the victim in jeopardy for further assaults. Furthermore, delays can impede the legal process because evidence is lost with time. Delays in the sequencing of collecting forensic evidence are important to the integrity of a case. Thus, the CSAAT-E clarifies the date and time of day of the assault, time lapse from assault to disclosure,

Box 1. Case study

Ms. G., age 65, was a widow and mother of one daughter. She had a high school education and a strong and uninterrupted work history up until the rape. Her health was good, with the exception of allergies, a recently diagnosed arthritic hip, and developing cataracts.

At about 3 PM, Ms. G. was exiting a toilet stall in a ladies' restroom at her work place when she was confronted with an assailant who pointed an ice pick to her throat. She was immobilized by the assailant tying her arms behind her back with a belt, tying a gag around her mouth, and taking her pantyhose and panties off her. She was digitally and vaginally penetrated. The sexual acts were multiple, prolonged, and painful due to the rapist having retarded ejaculation. She was also robbed of her wallet. After the assailant fled, she freed herself, left the area, and notified her supervisor. The police were called, and she was taken to a hospital for a forensic examination.

The SANE reported a stellate tear approximately 3 cm in length across the widest part and about 1 cm centrally above the urethral opening. There was also a small 1- to 1.5-cm tear in the posterior vagina at the introitus. There was bleeding from the vaginal area. The labia were swollen. Bruising was present, and small amounts of blood continued to ooze from the area. Lab tests: Vaginal smear indicated moderate red blood cells, white blood cells, epithelial cells, 4 + bacteria; no yeast or trichomonas seen. No chlamydia and no gonococcus were isolated. Forensic testing revealed DNA that was subsequently matched with an offender.

Subsequently, Ms. G's symptoms included decreased concentration, frequency of illnesses, extreme anxiety, panic attacks, nightmares, hypervigilance, and fear of return to work. Her health deteriorated, and she retired from her employment of 20 years. She was in counseling for 18 months and then moved to another state. She continued counseling by telephone with her therapist.

The crime was classified as a Primary Felony Rape. The assailant's intent was robbery, and he targeted a vulnerable environment. The victim was at the scene and was sexually assaulted as a situational second offense. The assailant used restraints found in the building (eg, black belt to tie her hands and a pink belt to gag her mouth).

Ms. G. worked with a police artist on a sketch of the assailant that was widely distributed around the business area. Several weeks later, a police officer noticed a loiterer at the building

where the rape had occurred. He matched the man to his police sketch and arrested him. In an affidavit, the assailant described how, 2 weeks before the rape, he consistently entered the
building through the front door on at least five occasions, rode
the elevator to various floors, surveyed the 16th and 17th floor,
and was never stopped by any security guards. When he saw
Ms. G. on the 17th floor, he returned to the elevator, went to the
16th floor where he stole some belts that were in boxes, and
returned to the 17th floor where he found Ms. G. in the bathroom.
After restraining, robbing, and raping her, he took the elevator
and exited the building without being stopped. The next day
he returned to the building to get food and to continue his criminal activities.

The criminal case was plea-bargained due to the DNA evidence
and the assailant's confession. A verdict in the civil suit was
awarded to the plaintiff.

time lapse from assault to evidence kit collection and examination, who the
disclosure was made to, and the victim's behavioral and physical indicators that
led to the discovery of the assault (Box 1).

Victim core elements

In addition to the items used in the original CSAAT (Table 1), the revised
CSAAT added questions about physical or mental limitations to show the
existence of these conditions before the assault. The critical elements subsumed
under the victim construct, pre-assault, are the following biopsychosocial
characteristics: physical and mental condition, race, ethnicity, gender, age, living situation, relationship to offender, and history of abuse. These factors
generate detailed information about patterns of functioning before and after
the assault. The post-assault biopsychosocial characteristics include mental
and physical functional status, disclosure of abuse, examination, response to
examination, severity of injury, and post-trauma response.

Nearly half of the victims in this study had some type of baseline physical
or mental disability that obscured disclosure or the investigation of a sexual
assault. As individuals age, they experience an increase in medical problems,
including cognitive and sensory impairment. Clinical and investigative expert's
report that markers of abuse mimic changes of aging and make the assessment
and prosecution of elder sexual abuse more complicated. For example, in
several cases in our study, the women had extensive bruising in the perineal
area that was initially attributed to perineum care. Further investigation showed

Table 1
Summary of revisions: Comprehensive Sexual Assault Assessment Tool

Original Comprehensive Sexual Assault Assessment Tool (CSAAT)	Revised Comprehensive Sexual Assault Assessment Tool for Elders (CSAAT-E)
Victim Core Elements	Victim Core Elements:
Characteristics: age, gender, race, marital status, education, occupation, primary language.	Characteristics: Existence (yes/no) of the condition prior to the assault
Forensic data:	1. History of interpersonal violence, sexual abuse, physical abuse
1. Physical: Height, weight, and vital signs; date and time of last consensual sex; condom used; urinated, defecated, vomited after assault; type of exam (direct visualization, bimanual exam speculum exam, colposcopic exam); photographs taken, evidence kit collected; tests for STD, sperm presence; Genital trauma, physical trauma; treatment provided (STD, urinary tract infection, other)	2. Presence of physical and mental disabilities
	3. Self Performance with activities of daily living
	4. Mental status: memory, sleep cycle, mood
	5. Diagnoses (Medical/Mental)
	Forensic data
2. Psychological: Victim's behavior during the exam and interview (controlled or expressive demeanor); seen by a counselor for Post Trauma assessment.	1. Physical: Severity of injury determined using the Abbreviated Injury Score (AIS).
	2. Psychological: Measure of SPAN instrument to measure startle, physiology, anger, numbness. Existence (yes/no) of the condition before the assault.
	3. Disposition following the exam: home, nursing home, medical admission, psychiatric admission, safe house/shelter, other
Offender Core Elements	Offender Core Elements
Characteristics: age, gender, race, marital status, education, unique features (i.e.; tattoos, facial/body hair), primary language, previous criminal record, number of offenders, use of drugs or alcohol; offender relationship to the victim	1. Characteristics: History of interpersonal violence, sexual abuse, physical abuse, presence of physical and/or mental limitations.
Method of approach, attack, and control: weapons (type), con, subterfuge, ploy, or blitz; use of gloves, bindings, telephone disabled, weapons; threatening methods of control (psychological coercion or physical force).	2. Relationship of the offender to the victim (stranger/acquaintance, unrelated care provider, incestuous, marital/partner, resident-to-resident, other
	3. Offender history of crime and drug abuse

Crime Core Elements

1. Date, time, and day of the week; location, type and sequence of sexual acts; number of offenders; single or multiple crimes; Victim's response to the offender (resistance and offenders reaction); presence of offender sexual dysfunction

2. Integrity of evidence (Offender took evidence from the scene; victim evidence not complete due to bathing, removal of cloths, etc.

Case Disposition Core Elements

1. Notification of police; offender (identified, arrested, charged, tried), plea bargain, guilty/not guilty

Crime Core Elements

1. Time lapse from a) assault to disclosure b) assault to exam, c) assault to investigation by police.

2. Location of the assault is specified as personal residence, nursing home, assisted living, other

3. Was an Evidence Kit collected (yes/no)?

4. Protective service involvement?

Case Disposition Core Elements

1. What was substantiated as a result of the investigation? (Sexual abuse, physical abuse, neglect, financial exploitation, self neglect, emotional abuse, nothing was substantiated, other).

2. Outcomes: (death, physical/mental problems)

3. Current status of the case (date): police notified, report filed, case closed, victim recanted, beyond statute of limitations, DA rejected, out of jurisdiction, false report, leads exhausted, pending DA review

4. Case inactivated: indicted, charged, convicted (plea, trial), sentenced.

Note: Variables from the original CSAAT are contained in the CSAAT-E, only additions are listed.

the bruising was due to sexual abuse. To compound matters in these cases, dementia and impaired communication from a stroke prevented early detection of the sexual abuse.

Causal relationships are obscured between injuries from sexual assault and injuries from a fall or other type of common procedure, such a perineum care for a dependent elder. Both sources of the injury can cause bruising. Because the cause of bruising can be attributed to a change in function of clotting mechanisms resulting in an increased susceptibility to bruising, doubt exists, and consequently it is difficult to establish objective relationships necessary for a successful prosecution. The CSAAT-E improves documentation of existing physical and mental conditions for the victim and the offender if only to show that certain conditions are risk factors or predispose victims to being vulnerable to attack or offenders to committing such crimes.

Special considerations are required for the frail elder with cognitive or sensory deficits. For example, an elder with compromised cognitive status might not be able to verbally articulate that he or she had been sexually assaulted. These elders can demonstrate clear signals of distress, which can be detected through identifying changes in patterns of verbal, behavioral, or physical expressions. Documentation of the functional status of victims is improved in the CSAAT-E and was considered an important core element for the database.

A reliable and valid measurement of trauma severity is essential to document outcomes from the assault. The original CSAAT did not have a scoring system to derive an injury severity score, nor did the instrument measure the psychologic impact of the trauma. Although the original instrument provided the necessary detail of the trauma to the sexual organs, there was less detail on other parts of the body. Close to 50% of the victims studied had vaginal trauma, and a third had other physical trauma. Severity scoring and estimating the probability of survival have potential applications for clinical and forensic practice. Determining the risk for injury and measurement of the physical impact on frail elders who were sexually assaulted are important revisions of the CSAAT-E.

The Abbreviated Injury Scale (AIS) and its derived injury severity scale quantify anatomic injury [14]. The AIS was incorporated into the revision of the CSAAT. The AIS is well established and has been used for many years to study the epidemiology and management of trauma [13]. The AIS was originally developed in 1971 by the American Association for Automotive Medicine, the Society of Automotive Engineers, and the American Medical Association to measure the extent of automobile accident injury [14]. The AIS uses specific codes for injuries and then attributes a score between 1 and 6 to each injury, classifying the injury as minor, moderate, serious, severe, critical, or fatal. An injury severity score can be computed from the sum of the squares of the AIS scores of the three most severe injuries. The computation has tested reliability for predicting survival in various populations [15]. The AIS and injury severity scoring system is a reliable and valid method for quantifying anatomic injury for the older adult population [16–18]. In one study, 38,707 seriously injured older adults were characterized using the AIS system in a retrospective secondary analysis of a statewide trauma data set from 1988 through 1997 [19]. The AIS was used to categorize injuries and compute an injury severity score.

The CSAAT-E includes a method for measuring the prevalence and patterns of post-traumatic stress symptomatology. Most of the victims studied did not have documentation of post-traumatic stress symptomatology. There is evidence that individuals experiencing traumatic events share similar patterns of responses [20–22]. However, little is known about the response of older adults to the trauma of sexual abuse. To document the psychologic trauma of sexual assault, we sought an instrument that was easy to use and sensitive to psychologic changes over time.

The SPAN scale is a four-item self-rated scale used in the diagnosis of post-traumatic stress disorder. SPAN is named for the four items: startle, physiologic arousal, anger, and numbness. The scale has correlated significantly with other accepted instruments of post-traumatic stress with a diagnostic accuracy of 88% [23]. Although there are many instruments to choose from to measure post-traumatic stress, the appeal of incorporating SPAN into the CSAAT-E was the parsimony of the four-item scale.

SPAN was developed from the Davidson Trauma Scale (DTS), which is a valid 17-item self-rating scale sensitive to measuring the effects of treatment [24]. Metzer-Brody et al [23], the authors of SPAN, believed a much shorter version of the DTS was possible because the DTS demonstrated a high level of item intercorrelation, with a Cronbach's alpha coefficient of 0.90. SPAN evaluates startle, physiologic arousal, anger, and numbness, which are symptoms specific to a post-traumatic stress diagnosis. Using SPAN in the CSAAT-E offers brevity, diagnostic accuracy, and the ability to distinguish between treatments of differing effectiveness. A limitation of SPAN is that it has not been psychometrically tested in the older adult population.

Finally, the revised CSAAT-E includes questions about the disposition of the victim after the examination. From this question, researchers are able to determine if a higher level of care was required after the assault. The question reads, "Following the exam, the victim is discharged to: home, nursing home, medical admission, psychiatric admission, safe house/shelter, or other."

Offender core elements

Few revisions were made to the offender core elements except to add information about a history of drug abuse; a previous criminal history; and a history of interpersonal violence, sexual abuse, physical abuse, or the presence of physical or mental limitations. The critical elements subsumed under the offender construct are the following biopsychosocial characteristics: physical and mental condition, race, ethnicity, gender, age, and living situation. The relationship of the offender to the victim is an important dimension for the older adult population. In many of the cases studied, the offender was known to the victim as a relative or caretaker.

The setting of the assault and relationship of the older adult to a perpetrator is an important dimension of evaluating risk factors. In our study, 43% of victims lived alone at home, and 38% of victims lived in nursing homes. Domestic and nursing home vulnerability to sexual assault for the older adult population is documented in the literature [9,25]. In both settings, the victim requires some level of assistance with physical or mental functioning. The type of living situation, functional status requiring aid from another person, and the relationship of the perpetrator to the victim were explicated in the CSAAT-E.

Our study showed that of the 125 elder sexual abuse cases, nursing home residents were more likely than non-nursing home residents to be older and physically and mentally disabled. The offenders for nursing home victims were more likely to be known to the victim or the victim's caretaker. These factors can change the approach to planning interventions that better protect vulnerable elders from perpetrators. In a study by the California Department of Justice, Certified Nursing Assistants (111,367) and Home Health Aids (36,314) criminal background checks were performed [26]. The study showed that 4.8% (10,130) of those employed had criminal histories. Certified Nursing Assistants and Home Health Aids predominantly care for the elderly in nursing homes and individual's homes. The expert group suggested a question be added to the CSAAT-E regarding a criminal record for the offender. Criminal background checks for all employees may be necessary to ensure safe environments for vulnerable elders.

Crime and case disposition core elements

The date, time, and day of the week and the location, type, and sequence of sexual acts were important elements in the original CSAAT along with the maintenance of the integrity of the evidence (eg, victim bathes or removes clothes before an evidentiary examination or the offender takes evidence from the scene of the crime). The CSAAT-E core data elements include essential crime information and information about the case disposition. Outcome measurement is essential for defining risk factors that inform appropriate treatment and preventative interventions. Not only are mortality and other adverse outcome measures important, but outcomes related to case disposition are required to determine the sensitivity of public systems to sexual assault crimes against older adults. The CSAAT-E includes greater detail about forensic evidence (eg, Was the evidence tampered with? Was the clinician performing the physical examination after the assault trained in the collection of forensic evidence?).

Other CSAAT changes included the need for better information about the closure of the assault case because often these victims are not believed or the cases are not substantiated or prosecuted. Furthermore, the experts hypothesized that early deaths were associated with a sexual assault but not identified as caused by injuries from the assault. Data correlating mortality and adverse outcomes among victims of elder sexual abuse are essential for identifying the consequences of this crime. Even if death is not a consequence of the sexual assault, worsening of physical and mental functioning can be a devastating outcome. The CSAAT-E includes questions about the circumstances of the case closure, the status of the victim, and prosecution detail.

Conclusion

Investigation and prosecution of an elder sexual crime presents unique challenges to the victim, the providers, and the criminal justice system. The medical, legal, and humanitarian costs of such crimes are immeasurable. Experts from this study anecdotally reported that victims often had serious complications or even death from being sexually assaulted, perhaps even more so than a younger cohort. Experts hypothesized that older adult sexual assault crimes result in an increased need for more costly health care, such as nursing home care or hospitalization. The personal suffering of the victim and their families must be considered along with a higher cost burden. Future research can examine such important dimensions.

When criminal conduct occurs, prompt detection, documentation, and referral are critical to permit the effective prosecution of cases. After a crime, all necessary elements must be proved beyond a reasonable doubt. Also, the perpetrator must be identified beyond a reasonable doubt. Finally, the competency of the victim to provide evidence must be determined [27]. These issues are important with the older adult victim who has physical or mental impairment. A reliable and valid national source of data about the sexual abuse of elders is essential to set standards from which prosecutors can base assumptions to secure the prosecution of offenders.

Summary

Understanding how intentional sexual injuries are inflicted on older adults is a growing concern as the population over 65 increases. This study contributes critical information to guide the identification of physical and psychologic markers of elder sexual abuse to be integrated by law enforcement and providers. Although there is still a great deal to learn, findings from this study will be used to educate health care professionals about elder sexual abuse, which we hope will in turn promote early detection. Building knowledge about unique psychologic and physical characteristics of sexually traumatized elders, outcomes (particularly exacerbation of comorbid conditions and death), and the effectiveness of interventions are essential for future research and policy development.

References

[1] Crowell NA, Burgess AW. Understanding violence against women. Washington, DC: National Academy Press; 1996.

[2] Criminal victimization 2000: changes 1989–2000 with trends 1993–2000. Available at: www.rainn.org/Linked%20files/NCVS%202000.pdf. Accessed June 14, 2004.

[3] Ramsey-Klawsnik H. Elder sexual abuse: preliminary findings. J Elder Abuse Negl 1991;3: 73–90.

[4] Teaster PB. A response to the abuse of vulnerable adults: the 2000 survey of state adult protective services. Washington, DC: The National Center on Elder Abuse; 2001.

[5] Gray MJ, Acierno R. Symptom presentation of older adult crime victims: description of a clinical sample. J Anxiety Disord 2002;16:299–309.

[6] Bachman R, Dillaway H, Lachs MS. Violence against the elderly. Res Aging 1998;20: 183–99.

[7] Falk B, Hasselt VB, Hersen M. Assessment of posttraumatic stress disorder in older victims of rape. J Clin Geropsychol 1997;3:157–71.

[8] Comijs HD, Pennix BW, Knipscheer KP, et al. Psychological distress in victims of elder mistreatment: the effects of social support and coping. J Gerontol Psychol Sci Soc Sci 1999; 54B:240–5.

[9] Teaster PB, Roberto KA, Duke JO, et al. Sexual abuse of older adults: preliminary findings of cases in Virginia. J Elder Abuse Negl 2000;12:1–17.

[10] Holt MG. Elder sexual abuse in Britain: preliminary findings. J Elder Abuse Negl 1993;5: 63–71.

[11] Burgess AW, Dowdell EB, Prentky RA. Sexual abuse of nursing home residents. J Psychosoc Nurs Ment Health Serv 2000;38:10–8.

[12] Burgess AW, Fawcett J. The comprehensive sexual assault assessment tool. Nurse Practitioner 1996;21;71–66, 78.

[13] Garthe E, States J, Mango N. Abbreviated injury scale unification: the case for a unified injury system for global use. J Trauma 1999;47:309–23.

[14] Wyatt JP, Beard D, Busuttil A. Quantifying injury and predicting outcome after trauma. Forensic Sci Int 1998;95:57–66.

[15] Osler T, Baker S, Long W. A modification of the injury severity score that both improves accuracy and simplifies scoring. J Trauma 1997;43:922–6.

[16] Boroos PL, Vanderschot P. Multiple trauma in elderly patients, factors influencing outcomes: importance of aggressive care. Injury 1993;38:10–8.

[17] Kilaru S, Garb J, Emhoff T. Long-term functional status and mortality of elderly patients with severe closed head injuries. J Trauma 1996;41:957–63.

[18] Zietlow SP, Capizzi PJ, Bannon MP. Multisystem geriatric trauma. J Trauma 1994;37:985–8.

[19] Richmond TS, Kauder D, Strumpf N, et al. Characteristics and outcomes of serious traumatic injury in older adults. J Am Geriatr Soc 2002;50:215–22.

[20] Burgess AW, Holstrom LL. Rape trauma syndrome. Am J Psychiatry 1974;131:981–6.

[21] Campbell JC. Battered women syndrome: a critical review. Violence Update 1990;1:10–1.

[22] Foa EB, Riggs DS, Gershuny BS. Arousal, numbing, intrusions: symptom structure of PTSD following assault. Am J Psychiatry 1995;152:116–20.

[23] Metzer-Brody S, Churchill E, Davidson JRT. Derivation of the SPAN, a brief diagnostic screening test for post-traumatic stress disorder. Psychiatry Res 1999;88:63–70.

[24] Davidson JRT, Book SW, Colket JT, et al. Assessment of a new self-rating scale for post-traumatic stress disorder. Psychol Med 1997;27:143–60.

[25] Burgess AW, Hanrahan NP. Issues in elder sexual abuse in nursing homes. Nurs Health Policy Rev 2004;3(1):5–17.

[26] Robison A. California Department of Justice certified nursing assistant and home health aid criminal background checks. (Summary of findings from a National Institute of Justice, grant no. 2001-IJ-CX-K015). In: Hanrahan N, editor. Boston: Chestnut Hill; 2000.

[27] Oreskovich MR, Howard JD, Copass MK. Geriatric trauma: injury patterns and outcome. J Trauma 1984;24:565–72.

CLINICS IN
GERIATRIC
MEDICINE

ELSEVIER
SAUNDERS

Clin Geriatr Med 21 (2005) 429–447

Community Approaches to Elder Abuse

Carmel B. Dyer, MD[a,b,c,*], Candace J. Heisler, JD[d],
Carrie A. Hill, BSW[c,e], Lucia C. Kim, MD, MPH[a,b,c]

[a]Department of Medicine, Baylor College of Medicine, 3601 N. MacGregor Way,
Houston, TX 77004, USA
[b]Geriatrics Program, Baylor College of Medicine, 3601 N. MacGregor Way, Houston, TX 77004, USA
[c]Texas Elder Abuse & Mistreatment (T.E.A.M.) Institute, 3601 N. MacGregor Way,
Houston, TX 77004, USA
[d]CJ Heisler & Associates, 134 Oxford Lane, San Bruno, CA 94066, USA
[e]Texas Department of Family and Protective Services, 5424 Polk Street, Houston, TX 77023, USA

The National Elder Abuse Incidence Study estimated that in 1996 at least one half million community-dwelling elders experienced abuse, neglect, or self-neglect [1]. A longitudinal study of a large cohort of community-dwelling older adults revealed Adult Protective Service (APS) use prevalence of 6.4% over an 11-year period [2]. Although other epidemiologic studies have estimated the prevalence of elder mistreatment (abuse, neglect, or exploitation) in the community in a variety of settings, experts agree that these reports represent only the tip of the iceberg and that elder abuse and neglect remain greatly hidden problems.

Elders in the community often experience the deterioration of their social network that may contribute to cognitive and functional decline [3], factors that have been linked to elder abuse and neglect in the community. The National Elder Abuse Incidence Study found that elders unable to care for themselves were at greater risk of experiencing abuse; approximately 60% of victims whose abuse was substantiated had some degree of mental impairment. Other risk factors for abuse and neglect in the community include poor social functioning as

---

* Corresponding author. Department of Medicine, Baylor College of Medicine, 3601 N. MacGregor Way, Houston, TX 77004.
   E-mail address: cdyer@bcm.tmc.edu (C.B. Dyer).

manifested by expressions of conflict with family or friends, social isolation, alcohol abuse, and psychiatric illness [4].

In the majority of states, health care professionals, such as licensed or registered nurses, physicians, and nurse's aides, are mandated reporters of elder abuse and neglect. Although physicians report only 0.6% to 2% of cases and nonphysician health care professionals report 11% to 26% of cases [5,6], physicians and other health care professionals are in a unique position to detect elder abuse and neglect and assess for the physical, mental, and medical needs of the elderly person. Physicians and other health care professionals are often the only noncaregivers with whom an older person has contact. Elder abuse and neglect often go undetected because of a lack of knowledge, denial of the problem, confounding problems related to aging, and the absence of uniform definitions [5].

Caring for elders living in the community who are abused or neglected requires collaboration of professionals from diverse disciplines. Elder abuse and neglect cases often pose multiple, complex issues that may be social, medical, ethical, legal, and financial in nature and that require expertise beyond that available from any single discipline [7]. Therefore, an interdisciplinary team effort is needed to effectively manage them. Depending on the type and work of the team, members may include a variety of professionals, such as physicians, nurses, social workers, APS caseworkers, law enforcement personnel, prosecutors, clergy, and representatives from financial institutions.

In this article, we discuss several types of teams and the issues they encounter when managing elder abuse and neglect in the community. The teams that are described include medical case management teams that focus on the medical and social aspects, legal intervention teams that address criminal and civil case development and the special legal and ethical issues that frequently arise, and APS teams that advocate for the elder's autonomy and liaise between elders in the community and services available to assist them. We discuss other specialized teams including the Fiduciary Abuse Specialist Teams (FAST) and Fatality Review teams (FRTs). We then discuss how a medical practitioner can respond to cases of elder abuse and neglect and the multiples resources available for elders in the community.

Duty to report

Although physicians have long been familiar with child abuse reporting requirements, the duty to report suspected elder abuse to legal entities is much less familiar. Medical ethics require that care be rendered to persons whether they abide by or break the law [8]. For the most part, patient–physician communications are considered confidential and not discoverable. Every state has a designated protective services agency to receive reports and assist older or vulnerable or frail adults. In all but six states (New York, Delaware, Wisconsin,

Colorado, and South Dakota) [6], physicians must report cases of elder mistreatment to these agencies. Although in 16 states, every citizen is a mandatory reporter [6], mandatory reporting laws generally apply to professionals who routinely encounter vulnerable populations, such as medical, mental heath, social service, and law enforcement personnel. In addition, every state provides for permissive reporting of suspected abuse or neglect by anyone. Although the specifics of reporting laws vary from state to state, failure to report is a punishable offense in 42 states [6]. Statutes are intended to encourage reporting, and, therefore, good faith reporters are immune from civil and criminal lawsuits. Protective services agencies must keep the identity of the reporter confidential.

Reporting allows states to measure the extent of the problem, to offer services to at-risk adults, to tailor delivery of social services to the needs of its citizens, and to identify and track perpetrators. The reportable conduct does not have to be criminal, and in most cases no criminal conduct has occurred. Most importantly, reporting provides access to a host of services that would not otherwise be available. These services are directly provided by or secured by caseworkers of APS agencies.

Adult protective services

History

Protective service agencies, including APS, are the public organizations responsible for investigating allegations of abuse, neglect, and exploitation of elderly and disabled adults. The problem of elder abuse in the community gained early recognition in the 1960s. A few states and local social service agencies began limited efforts to address it. The first federal government measures to address elder abuse came in Title XX of the Social Security Act of 1974. The Act gave individual states authorization to use Social Service Block Grant funds to protect the elderly persons in addition to children [9].

Although Title XX allowed individual protective service programs to expand, subsequent federal funding has failed to ensure adequate monies and legislation to allow APS programs to become uniform and well funded. APS programs often fall under the same agency umbrellas as Child Protective Services (CPS) and are forced to compete with CPS for funding and resources. APS does not receive the attention and community awareness that CPS commands. According to a 2002 white paper by the Senate Special Committee on Aging, federal funding appropriated for elder abuse totaled $153 million dollars; $520 million dollars were expended on violence against women programs; and $6.7 billion dollars were spent on child abuse prevention programs [9].

With minimal federal funding provided to support elder protective services programs, the states have had to appropriate money to fund these programs. The result has been wide variation in APS programs across the country. APS programs have differing policies, procedures, resources, and staffing. Agencies may be administered at the state, county, or local level.

All APS programs operate under the same philosophic principles. Core principles include advocating for each individual's constitutional right to autonomy, preserving the rights of individuals with capacity to make their own decisions, and selecting the least restrictive alternative among service options. The preservation of the family unit is also a priority. APS casework usually consists of case investigation, substantiation of one or more allegations, and intervention.

Adult Protective Services investigation

APS workers must depend on persons in the community to bring cases of abuse, neglect, or exploitation to their attention. Although there are legal protections for reporters, many cases are not reported. According to the National Elder Abuse Incidence Study [1], for every reported incident of elder abuse, neglect, exploitation, or self-neglect, approximately five are unreported. Most reports are of suspected self-neglect. Some of the reasons for failure to report include the lack of awareness of the existence or capabilities of APS, belief that reporting will compromise their relationship with the patient's family and that nothing will be done to improve the situation, fear of state involvement in the matter, concern that the reporter will face retaliation from the alleged perpetrator, and the desire to avoid the court process.

APS investigations are initiated by reports and proceed according to different policy-driven response times. An "emergency case," where there is an immediate danger to life and health, is ordinarily addressed within hours to a day. In non-emergency cases, and depending on the program, investigations begin anywhere from 1 to 14 days after the report is received. Some APS programs have 24-hour call centers and on-call staff. In other programs, the police or the emergency department staff address immediate needs until protective service workers can be contacted on the next business day.

Investigations include an interview with the client. In most states, APS workers are directed to attempt to interview the alleged perpetrator. They contact collateral sources for additional information about the client, including Social Security personnel, mental health professionals, primary care physicians, home health staff, family, friends, neighbors, financial institutions, and law enforcement. APS staff obtains and uses photographs of bruises/markings, hospital records, police reports, bank statements, canceled checks, and other forms of documentation as part of their investigations.

Confidentiality often is an obstacle for caseworkers attempting to obtain health and financial information. The recent Health Information Portability Accountability Act (HIPAA) has made obtaining information more difficult for APS caseworkers. Many states have statutes that mandate release of information and records to APS to assist them in their investigations. HIPAA regulations do not overturn existing state and federal laws, but confusion over HIPAA and its applications have meant that some organizations that should be providing records to APS are failing to do so.

Case substantiation

Workers usually have between 30 and 60 days to complete an investigation and determine the validity of an allegation. APS workers deem cases substantiated, unsubstantiated, or indeterminate. Some states require a preponderance of evidence standard to substantiate a case, whereas others require a higher degree of proof. At times there is limited objective evidence to support an allegation; workers must often weigh one person's word against another's and assess the credibility of those interviewed. Sometime there are not enough objective findings to make a determination. Cases are considered indeterminate when there is not enough evidence to prove or disprove the allegation.

At times, cases are not substantiated. In a small number of cases, the data collected do not support the allegation. On occasion, a false report is made, usually to embarrass or exact revenge on the client or the alleged perpetrator. This is not only a serious misuse of community resources, but in some states it is also a crime. Unsubstantiated cases are closed.

In a survey of state APS programs, performed by the National Association of Adult Protective Service Administrators, 41 states responded to a question concerning substantiation rates. The mean substantiation rate was calculated to be 48.4% and ranged from 2.2% in Florida to 100% in Indiana [6]. This wide variation may be due to differing definitions of a substantiated case and criteria for case investigation. After substantiation, caseworkers can develop intervention plans for their clients.

Adult Protective Service intervention

APS caseworkers can marshal a number of services to address client neglect, abuse, and other mistreatment. APS services are voluntary, and the client has the right to accept or decline them. APS interventions can be grouped into the following categories:

- Arranging for housing services, including emergency housing, cleaning services, home repairs, and home modification to meet the needs of persons with disabilities
- Obtaining medical services, including temporary medications, referral to health care for assessments, and assisting with application for health care benefits
- Addressing personal needs, including obtaining food delivery, applying for food stamps, and securing caretaker or other provider services
- Providing service coordination, such as short-term case management, providing linkage to other service groups

- Serving as a client advocate when family members are unavailable to interact with health professionals or make application for community programs
- Implementing legal interventions, such as guardianship, involuntary mental health commitments, and emergency removals (referred to differently depending on the state)

Legal interventions are the most restrictive actions an APS worker can use. They are used only when all other less restrictive alternatives have failed or are clearly inappropriate. Although there is variation between states regarding available legal options, typically each requires the involvement of medical practitioners before or after the initial action is taken. Physicians are often involved when an adult's decision-making capacity is an issue. Questions may arise when a client refuses needed services or remains in unsafe situations. APS seek the assistance of an agency attorney to bring the matter to the attention of the local court where the judge decides the person's legal competency.

If adults suffering from mental illness or cognitive impairment are at immediate risk of hurting themselves or others or require medical attention but have refused to receive it because they lack capacity to understand the consequence of the decision, APS caseworkers can obtain mental health warrants or emergency removal orders. Emergency removal orders (the name for this varies from state to state) usually require judicial approval and authorize temporary involuntary admission into a psychiatric or medical hospital. The implementation of either of these frequently results in the ultimate pursuit of legal guardianship.

Legal guardianship (also called conservatorship in a few states) is the permanent removal of a person's right to make his or her own decisions. It is implemented in situations where clients are no longer able to manage their personal or financial affairs and have not designated a surrogate decision maker. Although it is the most restrictive alternative, its requirements of judicial involvement and oversight and due process protections for wards and conservatees are intended to reduce opportunities for misuse and abuse [10]. Where guardians are needed but no responsible family members or friends are available, in some state or regions, APS workers assume this role. In other sites, social services caseworkers, private guardians and conservators, public guardians, or lawyers may be appointed. Usually, a guardianship results in placement in a facility setting due to supervision requirements or medical condition that prompted the APS worker to seek guardianship in the first place.

Myths and misperceptions about Adult Protective Services

Although caseworkers conduct investigations, APS has no law enforcement authority. Some equate APS workers with hospital social workers, but not all APS workers are social workers, and not all have bachelor's degrees. There is a fear that APS involvement always results in the removal of older persons from their homes and their placement in institutions. Legal interventions are used in only 7% of cases nationally. Some believe that APS workers can force nonadherent clients to accept services. However, as agents of the state their authority is defined by statute, and under existing laws, APS workers cannot impose interventions on persons with the capacity to make decisions.

The need for multidisciplinary collaborations

A critical issue facing protective services and its ability to impose services and interventions on an unwilling adult is a determination of his or her decision-making capacity. Although the APS caseworker is charged with assessing capacity, there are no validated and reliable instruments designed for use by nonmedical professionals. When APS workers suspect that a client lacks capacity, they must determine if the client understands the consequences of their decisions. Workers must evaluate if there are any indications of mental illness, dementia, or other cognitive impairment, notwithstanding the reality that persons with early and even moderate dementia have preserved social skills that make it especially difficult to accurately assess their capacity [11–13]. Some persons, especially those with high intelligent quotients or who are highly educated, maintain excellent verbal skills while lacking insight, good judgment, or the physical ability to care for themselves in a safe manner. In such "gray" cases, the determination of capacity can be difficult for highly trained and skilled physicians. Such determinations are fraught with difficulties for APS workers who are differently skilled and trained.

Medically based community resources, such as medical case management teams (described below), are essential to making such determinations and providing good care to clients [14]. Where available, APS staff turn to geriatricians, generalists, psychiatrists, or other medical professionals to formally assess the client's ability to understand the consequences of decisions and to advise in diagnosing and treating existing medical conditions. In some communities, qualified and willing medical experts to assess capacity are not always available, so APS must make these difficult assessments without them.

The rest of this article addresses the many disciplines that interact with mistreated elders and the formal and informal community-based collaborations that have formed to better identify, intervene, and prevent elder abuse.

Medical case management teams

For the last 20 years, geriatricians and gerontologists have been performing comprehensive geriatric assessment (CGA) and intervention in their frail patients. CGA includes assessments of social situation, functional status, and health [15,16]. CGA uses an interdisciplinary approach because members of no single discipline posses all the skills required to meet the needs of frail older persons. Numerous studies have demonstrated the benefits of CGA and intervention to hospitalized, institutionalized, and community-dwelling elders [17–19]. It is not surprising, then, that this interdisciplinary approach would be applied to mistreated elders who are frail and also vulnerable.

History

In response to a Massachusetts law enacted in 1980, a medical interdisciplinary case management team was formed at the Beth Israel Hospital in Massachusetts. The purpose of this team is to provide consultation and support to hospital staff, assist in a multidimensional evaluation of older patients where abuse is suspected, and develop treatment plans. The team, composed of a physician, nurses, and social workers, meets weekly to discuss referred cases. The team also educates hospital staff about identification and intervention in elder abuse [20]. Another hospital-based team formed in the 1998 at Mount Sinai Hospital in New York to detect elder mistreatment in hospitalized patients and ". . .to assist them in attaining compensation, and to provide counseling, support, advocacy and referral" [21].

Physicians and medical teams throughout the United States have been and are informally collaborating with APS in their communities. In the mid-1990s, geriatric medicine teams began to formally collaborate with Adult Protective Services at Baylor College of Medicine in Houston, Texas, at the University of California at Irvine in Orange County, at the Robert Woods Johnson Medical School in New Jersey, and at Hennepin Medical Center in Minnesota [22]. These teams address all forms of elder abuse and self-neglect. Although each educates trainees from a variety of disciplines about elder abuse intervention, differences in setting, funding, and the local needs of APS make each team unique.

The medical case management team generally cares for the more medically complex victims, especially self-neglectors. This team usually operates within a health care system and draws on the expertise of a full range of medical specialists. Its membership looks like a geriatric interdisciplinary team, with members from geriatric medicine, nursing, social work, and other health care fields, but also includes APS workers and may include law enforcement officers, attorneys, and victim advocates. Often ethicists, forensic psychiatrists, and members of other medical disciplines are called to provide consultation.

The work of the medical case management team

The medical case management team generally receives referrals from APS, although law enforcement, medical examiners, prosecutors, and others may refer cases. Despite variation in local needs and the capabilities and interests of members, the work of these teams is similar and usually takes place in three phases. The first phase is the investigation or assessment that a member from the referring agency performs. In the next phase, a comprehensive geriatric assessment is conducted by the medical team, and assessment or investigations as needed are undertaken by team members from other disciplines. The third phase is the interdisciplinary team meeting, where all the participating members craft a joint intervention plan. In the same way that interdisciplinary geriatric medicine case conferences help team members learn about each other's disciplines, divides the work, prevents duplication of effort, and enables the development of innovative and effective care plans, so do elder mistreatment medical case management teams provide benefit to patients, the participants, and their organizations. Finally, the intervention plan is performed (Fig. 1).

Assessment

House calls.   House calls are often a major function of elder mistreatment case management teams in situations where patients refuse to leave their homes. These patients may be fearful, ashamed of their circumstances, or unable to physically leave the dwelling, and a house call may be the only way for that patient to receive care. House calls afford the clinician a clearer view of how the patient functions in his or her own environment and makes detection of some forms of abuse, such as self-neglect or financial exploitation, easier. The diagnosis of hoarding or Diogenes syndrome, an extreme form of self-neglect, is diagnosed by visual inspection of the patient's living situation.

Common diagnoses.   The medical team performs a comprehensive geriatric assessment regardless of the setting where the evaluation takes place. Victims of elder mistreatment and self-neglect most often are diagnosed with dementia, depression, psychosis, alcohol abuse, and loss of executive function [23–25]. Much of the work of the medical case management team involves assessment and intervention on behalf of patients who are experiencing cognitive decline

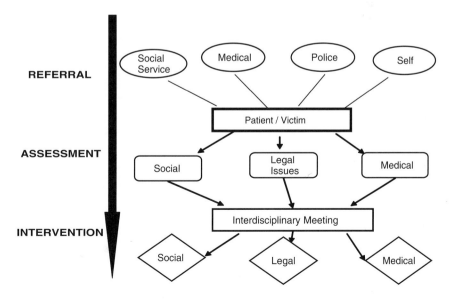

Fig.1. Sample medical case management team process.

leading to frailty and the inability to provide their own care. In some cases, cognitive decline affects the patient's judgment, resulting in their refusal of much-needed APS or medical interventions. Because APS workers are guided by the principle of self-determination and have different expertise from health care professionals, they may be persuaded by articulate or impassioned pleas of clients who wish to remain in questionable situations. It is in these cases that the physician's expertise in assessing decision-making capacity is critical to the team's evaluation.

Case management team interventions. After multidimensional comprehensive geriatric assessment, the interdisciplinary team members meet for case review. The group discusses the diagnoses or findings determined from the comprehensive evaluation. The members then craft appropriate intervention plans. Patients suffering from physical abuse receive treatment for their injuries. Self-neglectors or victims of caregiver neglect may (and frequently do) require intervention for neurocognitive or affective disorders. Treatment is provided for any identified reversible disorders. Physical and occupational therapists may treat to restore function. The medical professionals work with members of the team from various disciplines to craft comprehensive interventions plans and jointly participate in decisions regarding living situations. Medical case management team interventions include the following:

- Treating or curing disease states. These teams work to improve cognitive status by providing medication and mental retraining, improve functional status by prescribing therapy or assistive devices, treat behavioral disorders with appropriate medical and environmental modifications, and adjust/ monitor complex medication regimens.
- Prevention of deterioration by monitoring health status and responding to acute physical and mental changes, improving nutrition, and recommending appropriate modifications to living situations
- Educating patients about their disease states and requirements for improved health and training caregivers
- Providing palliative care at the end of life by controlling pain and symptoms

Finally, on occasion medical examiners, physicians, nurses, and other health professionals may be needed to offer expert testimony in criminal and civil proceedings.

Legal intervention teams

Although APS agencies address the social and functional issues faced by mistreated elders and medical case management teams address health, function, and social issues, it is the justice system that must address the legal concerns. Mistreated elders may be victims of physical abuse, criminal neglect, sexual assault, and intimate partner violence, and they need protection. Experts to address financial management, probate and guardianships, other legal issues, housing, and more are needed. Specialized teams exist to deal with these serious legal issues.

The criminal justice system

The criminal justice system includes law enforcement officers and prosecutors. Its role is to stop criminal conduct, protect individual victims and society from criminal acts, hold offenders accountable, make victims whole by restoring their personal losses, and rehabilitate perpetrators [26]. The role of law enforcement in elder abuse is assessment, enforcement, support, and referral [27]. Law enforcement officers conduct investigations, determine if crimes have occurred, interview witnesses, collect evidence, and, when appropriate, make arrests. The prosecution function focuses on deciding whether to bring criminal charges and the presentation of cases in court, including the production of witnesses and evidence and sentencing recommendations [28]. Criminal justice interventions include the following:

- Holding offenders accountable by initiating charges, prosecuting cases on behalf of the community, prosecution and law enforcement working together during investigations, seeking increased bail or remand, conducting grand jury investigations, issuing subpoenas, and obtaining convictions, seeking case appropriate conditions of probation, and filing motions seeking sanctions for violations of probation or failure to pay restitution
- Assisting victims by providing information about the legal system, obtaining court orders, seeking orders of restitution, presenting victim impact information at sentencing, and appearing at parole hearings to resist early release
- Responding to crime reports by collecting evidence, conducting forensic evidence examinations, identifying perpetrators, and arresting offenders
- Obtaining court orders, such as arrest and search warrants, and other orders to protect victims (where permitted)
- Increasing safety by seizure of weapons, performing welfare checks, and accompanying various professionals and team members on house calls/ home visits
- Obtaining medical assistance for injured or ill victims and psychiatric care for mentally disturbed persons

Criminal prosecution teams

There are a variety of criminal justice teams operating throughout the United States. These can be led by law enforcement, such as domestic violence response teams in which an officer works with a victim advocate to respond to cases of domestic violence, including cases involving elderly parties. The officer investigates crimes, collects evidence, and develops cases for possible prosecution while the advocate meets with the victim to address his or her immediate safety and other concerns. In Rapid Response Teams, investigators from a law enforcement agency or prosecutors office respond with APS caseworkers to reports of elder abuse. The caseworker investigates allegations of abuse and focuses on client needs and substantiation of elder abuse allegations while the investigator attempts to determine if a crime has occurred and, if so, to protect and secure remaining victim assets.

In some communities, the prosecutor works with various professionals and, upon receipt of a report of possible elder abuse, selects appropriate team members to investigate the matter and build the case for prosecution. One such team operates in the United States' Attorney's Office in Washington, DC. In other prosecutors offices, significant prosecution units have been created. These work closely with a variety of professionals including law enforcement, APS, health care providers, and others to address elder abuse allegations [29,30].

The civil justice system

Members of the civil justice system, including family, estate planning, tax, and probate lawyers, can pursue an array of legal remedies aimed at protecting victims, securing and restoring assets, assessing responsibility, and appointing surrogate decision makers. In the elder abuse arena, civil courts can issue a variety of protective orders, adjudicate lawsuits, issue emergency removal orders, order involuntary mental health placements, create guardianships, secure accountings, and order assets be frozen to protect remaining assets and estates.

Civil justice interventions include the following:

- Seeking court orders and guardianships to protect clients
- Initiating lawsuits on behalf of clients for such causes of action as theft, assault and battery, conversion, breach of contract, and negligence
- Advanced planning, including powers of attorney and trust

Fiduciary Abuse Specialist Teams

FASTs are an example of a civil justice–focused team; the purpose of a FAST is to develop financial exploitation cases. Teams are staffed by law enforcement officers, prosecutors, private and public interest attorneys, public and private conservators, bankers, securities and real estate brokers, APS workers, members of the Long Term Care Ombudsman Program, and experts in finances, insurance, care management, probate, gerontology, geriatrics, and psychiatry [31]. These partnerships of professionals volunteer their time to review cases and facilitate comprehensive service delivery [32]. The first FAST was established in Los Angeles County in 1993 [33].

As the benefits of the model have been identified, other FASTs have been created so that there are teams operating throughout California, parts of Oregon, and elsewhere. An innovative aspect of the Oregon team is its recruitment of volunteer, retired employees of financial institutions and analysts to analyze evidence and assist law enforcement and prosecutors in building financial exploitation criminal cases. Teams may also advocate for legislative reform, educate the community, and train professionals [32].

Other community-based approaches

Other types of collaborations have evolved to address different aspects of elder mistreatment. These include code enforcement teams, fatality review teams, and victim advocacy programs. Medical professionals can participate in any of these teams.

Code enforcement team

Code enforcement teams inspect locations and facilities where there are reported public nuisances or recurring reports of inadequate care. Team membership is drawn from regulatory and licensing agencies, law enforcement, fire services, pest control authorities, building inspectors, and investigators from offices of state attorneys general, city attorneys, and county counsel. Drawing on the expertise and authority of many officials, teams conduct unannounced inspections to identify dangerous, illegal, or unsanitary sites. If needed, they pursue administrative and licensing actions or file civil or criminal lawsuits to obtain improvements, clean up problematic locations, seek changes in procedures or management, or secure the closure of a facility. Teams may operate at the local or state level. Examples of state-level teams are those in Offices of the Attorney General in California and Florida that inspect problematic elder care facilities.

Fatality review teams

Elder abuse FRTs, a recent development in elder abuse, are often modeled on child and domestic violence death review teams. Their role is to review deaths of older persons that are believed to have resulted from elder abuse to assess systemic responses, such as problems with service delivery, and identify prevention strategies [31]. Some FRTs review cases to determine if prosecution should be considered. This team requires participation by the medical examiner or coroner. FRTs may recommend legislative changes, adoption of new policies by agencies, and elder abuse training. These teams operate in various locations across the country, including San Diego, Sacramento, and Orange County, California; Harris County, Texas; and Portland, Maine.

Victim advocacy organizations

Advocacy is an encompassing term that covers many different private and public agencies and organizations that serve victims of abuse and mistreatment.

Some organizations assist victims of domestic violence and sexual assault. Some serve elder abuse victims, and some serve all crime victims. Advocates may be community based or part of victim-witness assistance program associated with the criminal justice system. Many have special legally protected confidential relationships with their clients. Their services are voluntary and generally operate on an empowerment model in which programs and resources are offered to a victim who decides which, if any, are appropriate for his or her situation. Available services may include providing legal advocacy and assistance; helping with emergency shelter and new housing; obtaining health care services; coordinating support groups; applying for financial benefits; obtaining other emergency and longer-term services; and assisting with recovery from the physical, emotional, and financial effects of their victimizations.

How the practitioner can respond

With the range of possible interventions and the complex client needs that must be met by medical and legal professionals and others, collaboration with other disciplines may be more effective. The following is a case example of how an interdisciplinary medical case management team handles a case of care-giver neglect.

A 77-year-old woman, Mrs. R.L. was released from the hospital after intravenous treatment of lower extremity cellulitis; lacerations caused by her pet cat had become infected. She was also diagnosed with hypothyroidism and was begun on replacement therapy. At discharge, the physician wrote orders for a home health nurse to visit the patient.

Two days after discharge, the nurse went to Mrs. R.L.'s home and discovered the patient's home piled high with trash and rotting food. There were 10 cats roaming the premises. During an examination, the nurse met the patient's son who was intoxicated and shouting from his bedroom. The patient was lying in a bed without a sheet, wearing a soiled diaper and urine-soaked clothing. The nurse called the physician and reported the case to APS.

An APS caseworker went to Mrs. R.L.'s home the next day and confirmed that the environment was unclean and unsafe and that the patient was being neglected. The patient's son was threatening to the worker and was concerned that his mother would be removed from her home. The APS worker found evidence that the son was cashing Mrs. R.L.'s social security checks and using them to buy alcohol. The APS worker spoke to the neighbors who told her that Mrs. R.L.'s son had recently been incarcerated for assault with a deadly weapon. The neighbor confirmed that the son often yelled at his mother and threatened to leave her.

APS substantiated two allegations: caregiver neglect and financial exploitation. They consulted the medical elder abuse team in their community and requested that they make a house call to evaluate the patient. The team carefully orchestrated the house call. Based on the history of a threatening son, the medical team called the police and requested that an officer accompany them on the visit. The protective services lawyer was notified that an emergency removal order might be needed. A social worker and physician from the medical team went to Mrs. R.L.'s home and verified the nurse's findings. In addition, they discovered that the patient had multiple flea bites, was lethargic, and had a temperature of 95.7°F. Her mini-mental state score was 20, and the Confusion Assessment Method test was positive for delirium. The team suspected that the patient had hypothyroidism and informed the patient that she needed to go to a hospital for immediate attention. When the physician spoke to the patient and provided a detailed explanation of the risks of not being treated, the patient refused hospitalization.

The medical team contacted the APS attorney and indicated that Mrs. R.L. required emergency medical treatment. The attorney obtained a court order for Mrs. R.L.'s emergency removal from her home. Paramedics were called to transport her to the hospital where she was diagnosed with a urinary tract infection and a markedly elevated thyroid simulating hormone. After treatment, her mental status improved (MMSE of 25). She acknowledged that her son had a drinking problem but asked to return to her home to live with him. The medical team suspected that she had diminished decision-making capacity; this finding was confirmed by neuropsychologic testing.

An interdisciplinary team meeting was held. The APS worker reported that she had located the patient's daughter who was living out of state. Once informed of her mother's situation, the daughter was willing to become her mother's guardian. She asked that Mrs. R.L. move into her home. The physician, social workers, and nurses agreed that the patient would be safe in the community in her daughter's home and did not require nursing home placement. The patient's daughter applied to become her mother's guardian, and, over the son's opposition, the judge granted custody to the daughter. The son was arrested on a parole violation when a gun was found in the home by police officers; he is now incarcerated. His mother lives in a comfortable home and is receiving the medical care she needs.

This case is an illustration of how an interdisciplinary collaboration can be effective in a difficult and complex situation. The APS worker, police officers, physician, nurses, social workers, paramedics, a lawyer, and a judge participated in the intervention. The interdisciplinary team was able to coordinate a multiphase intervention that achieved the overarching goals of stopping the abuse, holding the offender accountable, improving the quality of life for the victim, and protecting the local community from the abusive son.

The involvement of these and other systems was necessary because cases like this are so complex and multifaceted that the response of a single system is not effective in addressing the problem. In the same way that geriatric teams evolved to meet the complex needs of frail elders, multidisciplinary elder mistreatment intervention teams have evolved to provide more comprehensive and effective interventions.

Other resources

In addition to protective service workers, medical professionals, and members of the civil and criminal justice systems, the assistance of members from other disciplines is required to design the most appropriate intervention plan. Professionals from a variety of community-based agencies can contribute to the work of elder mistreatment teams. They bring their unique perspectives and may offer different interventions. They can serve as resource personnel and are often asked to participate in the types of teams described previously on continuing or ad hoc bases. Some of the resources that may be helpful to elder mistreatment casework in the community described below.

Area Agencies on Aging were established under the Older Americans Act in 1973 and are located in every community. They provide a host of services that would be helpful in developing intervention plans. They provide information and access services (eg, health insurance counseling), community-based services (eg, adult day care), in-home services (eg, homemakers and Meals-on-Wheels), assistance with housing (eg, locating assisted living facilities or foster care), and support of elder rights (eg, legal assistance) [34].

Local women's shelters or centers house experts in the intervention of domestic violence and intimate partner violence involving younger women. Some centers may have staff with the expertise to deal with these same problems in elderly patients. Alternatively, the center staff could work with a medical case management team to adapt the techniques known to help younger women to the needs of older patients. Domestic violence intervention in elderly persons requires a specialized approach, and members of a medical case management teams may want to consult experts before proceeding.

The National Center for Elder Abuse (NCEA) is funded through the Administration on Aging [35]. They have a wealth of resources including national and state statistics. They have a training library and track elder mistreatment educational conferences for the entire United States. They have commissioned several studies, and two recent documents could be helpful to in communities that are developing or wish to develop a community-based response to elder mistreatment. They are "A National Look at Multidisciplinary Teams" [33] and Multidisciplinary Elder Abuse Prevention Teams: A New Generation [31].

The Clearinghouse for Abuse Neglect of the Elderly (CANE) is located at the University of Delaware and is funded by the NCEA. This archive is the nation's largest and includes published research, training resources, government documents, and other sources on elder abuse. The CANE collection is computerized, and interested parties can perform text searches. CANE has nearly 5000 holdings. The staff has compiled 12 bibliography series with annotated references; of particular interest is the series entitled "The Health Care System: Addressing Elder Mistreatment from July 2003" [36].

The National Clearinghouse on Abuse in Late Life was established by the Wisconsin Coalition Against Domestic Violence in 1999 with funding from the

Department of Justice's Office on Violence Against Women. The staff of this national organization has expertise in program development, policy and technical assistance, and training. They have assembled a directory of services that "contains nationwide resources, state domestic violence coalitions, state sexual assault coalitions, state adult protective services offices, elder shelters and support groups tailored to older women" [37].

The American Bar Association Commission on Law and Aging features a host of resources including legal guides, online brochures, and toolkits. Their literature provides advice to consumers and lawyers. This group cosponsors the National Law and Aging conference and has expertise in a number of issues, including planning for incapacity, guardianship, elder abuse, health care decision-making, pain management, and end-of-life care [38].

Summary

The role of medical professionals who address community elder abuse, like that for treating patients in hospitals or other outpatient settings, is to screen for elder mistreatment, diagnose overt or underlying disease states, and provide appropriate treatment while considering the patient's medical, social, functional, financial, and legal needs. This requires heightened awareness of elder mistreatment; knowledge of the historic and physical findings; ascertainment of collateral history; complete documentation of findings; and collaboration with members of other disciplines, including law and protective service. Physicians and other medical professionals, especially members of geriatric interdisciplinary teams, are well suited to collaborate and develop case management teams. Medical professionals can provide clinical care while training others and conducting research.

A number of elder mistreatment team models have formed. Their precise membership, focus, and goals vary based on the defined needs of the community in which they operate. Some focus on particular cases, whereas others review systems' responses to identify gaps in service and system weaknesses. Geriatricians and other gerontology professionals serve on all these teams. Elder abuse is a complex and multifaceted problem whose impact is felt by many different systems. Victims and their families frequently are served by multiple systems simultaneously. Systems responses may be inconsistent, philosophically at odds, and not comprehensive, but an effective intervention must recognize and understand other potential involved systems may be and what they do. In some places, the medical professional can play a critical role in improving their own and other systems' responses in an elder abuse matter.

Just as pediatricians championed the fight against child abuse in 1970s and 1980s, so can geriatricians and all health professionals who care for older persons become champions in the twenty-first century's fight against elder mistreatment.

References

[1] The National Center on Elder Abuse. American Public Human Services Association. The National Elder Abuse Incidence Study: final report. Washington, DC: Administration for Children and Families & Administration on Aging, US Department of Health and Human Services; 1998.

[2] Lachs M, Williams C, O'Brien S, et al. Older adults: an 11-year longitudinal study of adult protective service use. Arch Intern Med 1996;156:449–53.

[3] Yeh SC, Liu YY. Influence of social support on cognitive function in the elderly. BMC Health Serv Res 2003;3:9.

[4] Shugarman LR, Fries BE, Wolf RS, et al. Identifying older people at risk of abuse during routine screening practices. J Am Geriatr Soc 2003;51:24–31.

[5] Rosenblatt DE, Cho KH, Durance PW. Reporting mistreatment of older adults: the role of the physician. J Am Geriatr Soc 1996;44:65–70.

[6] A response to the abuse of vulnerable adults: the 2000 survey of state adult protective services. Available at: www.elderabusecenter.org/pdf/research/apsreport030703.pdf. Accessed December 15, 2004.

[7] Quinn MJ, Tomita SK. Elder abuse and neglect: causes, diagnoses and intervention strategies. New York: Springer; 1997.

[8] The American Medical Association's Declaration of Professional Responsibility. Available at: www.ama-assn.org/ama/pub/category/7491.html. Accessed December 15, 2004.

[9] Protecting America's seniors: a history of elder abuse and neglect from the United States Senate, Special Committee on Aging; 2002.

[10] Keith PM, Wacker RR. It is hard to guard the aged: role strain of male and female guardians. J Gerontol Social Work 1993;21:41–58.

[11] Volicer L, Ganzini L. Health professionals' views on standards for decision-making capacity regarding refusal of medical treatment in mild Alzheimer's disease. J Am Geriatr Soc 2003;51: 1270–4.

[12] Marson DC, Ingram KK, Cody HA, et al. Assessing the competency of patient's with Alzheimer's disease under different legal standards: a prototype instrument. Arch Neurol 1995; 52:949–54.

[13] Marson DC, Earnst KS, Jamil F, et al. Consistency of physician's legal standard and personal judgments of competency in patients with Alzheimer's disease. J Am Geriatr Soc 2000; 48:911–8.

[14] Dyer CB, Silverman E, Nguyen T, et al. The special case of elder abuse. In: Mezey MD, Cassell CK, Bottrell M, Hyer K, Howe JL, Fulmer T, editors. Ethical patient care: a casebook for geriatric health care teams. Baltimore: The Johns Hopkins University Press; 2002. p. 151–65.

[15] Abrams WB, Beers MH, Berkow R. Comprehensive geriatric assessment. In: Abrams WB, Beers MH, Berkow R, editors. The Merck Manual of Geriatrics. 2nd edition. Whitehouse Station (NJ): Merck Research Laboratories, Merck & Co., Inc.; 1995. p. 224–35.

[16] Siu AL, Reuben DB, Moore AA. Comprehensive geriatric assessment. In: Hazzard WR, Bierman EL, Blass JP, editors. Principles of geriatric medicine and gerontology. New York: McGraw-Hill; 1994. p. 202–12.

[17] Stuck AE, Aronow HU, Steiner A, et al. A trial of annual in-home comprehensive geriatric assessment for elderly people living in the community. N Engl J Med 1995;333:1184–9.

[18] Hendriksen C, Lund E, Stromgard E. Consequences of assessment and intervention among elderly people: a three-year randomized controlled trial. Br Med J (Clin Res Ed) 1984;289: 1522–4.

[19] Applegate WB, Miller ST, Graney MJ, et al. A randomized, controlled trial of a geriatric assessment unit in a community rehabilitation hospital. N Engl J Med 1990;322:1572–8.

[20] Matlaw JR, Spence DM. The hospital elder assessment team: a protocol for suspected cases of elder abuse and neglect. JEAN 1994;6:23–7.

[21] Kahan FS, Paris BE. Why elder abuse continues to elude the health care system. Mt Sinai J Med 2003;70:62–8.

[22] Heath JM, Dyer CB, Kerzner LJ, et al. Four models of medical education about elder mistreatment. Acad Med 2002;77:1101–6.

[23] Dyer CB, Goins AM. The role of the interdisciplinary geriatric assessment in addressing self-neglect of the elderly. Generations 2000;24:23–7.

[24] Dyer CB, Pavlik VN, Murphy KP, et al. The high prevalence of depression and dementia in elder abuse or neglect. J Am Geriatr Soc 2000;48:205–8.

[25] Abrams RC, Lachs M, McAvay G, et al. Predictors of self-neglect in community-dwelling elders. Am J Psychiatry 2002;159:1724–30.

[26] Heisler CJ. The role of the criminal justice system in elder abuse cases. JEAN 1991;3:5–33.

[27] Payne BK. Understanding differences in opinion and 'facts' between ombudsmen, police chiefs, and nursing home directors. JEAN 2001;13:61–77.

[28] Office for Victims of Crime's New Directions from the Field. Victims' rights and services for the 21st Century. Washington, DC: United States Department of Justice, Office of Justice Programs; 1998.

[29] Greenwood P. Elder abuse: a statewide perspective. Prosecutor's brief. California District Attorneys Assoc Q J 1999;XX1:5–6, 26–7.

[30] Rohn AL. A multi-disciplinary approach to elder abuse prosecution. Prosecutor's brief. California District Attorneys Assoc Q J 1999;XX1:7–8, 30–31.

[31] Nerenberg L. Multidisciplinary elder abuse prevention teams: a new generation. Available at: www.elderabusecenter.org/default.cfm. Accessed December 15, 2004.

[32] Allen JV. Financial abuse of elders and dependent adults: the FAST (Fiduciary Abuse Specialist Team) approach. JEAN 2000;12:85–91.

[33] Nerenberg L. A national look at multidisciplinary teams. Available at: www.elderabusecenter.org/default.cfm.

[34] National Association for Area Agencies on Aging. Available at: www.n4a.org/aboutn4a.cfm.

[35] National Center on Elder Abuse. Available at: www.elderabusecenter.org/default.cfm.

[36] Clearinghouse on Abuse and Neglect of the Elderly. Available at: www.elderabusecenter.org/default.cfm?p=cane.cfm.

[37] National Clearinghouse on Abuse in Late Life. Available at: www.ncall.us.

[38] American Bar Association's Legal Commission on Law and Aging. Available at: www.abanet.org/aging/mission.html.

ELSEVIER
SAUNDERS

CLINICS IN
GERIATRIC
MEDICINE

Clin Geriatr Med 21 (2005) 449–457

Elder Abuse, Neglect, and Exploitation: Policy Issues

Kathleen Quinn[a],*, Holly Zielke, MA[b]

[a]*1315 Noble Avenue, Springfield, IL 62704, USA*
[b]*Elder Abuse Program, Illinois Department on Aging, 100 W. Randolph Street, Suite 10-350,
Chicago, IL 60601, USA*

Elder abuse has a long and confusing history as a public policy issue. First emerging in the 1970s as "granny bashing" in British publications, it was brought to the forefront in the United States at a 1978 congressional sub-committee hearing on family violence [1]. This was followed by a 1979 United States House of Representatives Select Committee on Aging hearing in 1979 and a bill—the Prevention, Identification and Treatment of Adult Abuse Act—introduced by Rep. Rose Oakar in 1980, that would have provided funds to states for adult protective services (APS) [2]. In 1985, Rep. Claude Pepper, an outspoken champion for seniors, stated that "Congress should act immediately to assist the states in preventing, identifying and assisting our nation's elder abuse victims" [3].

Despite continued findings and hearings, no federal elder abuse legislation has passed, with the exception of Title VII of the Older Americans Act, which provides just over $5 million for the nation to increase public awareness of the issue [4]. Because these funds are distributed by interstate formulas to each state's unit on aging, and then by intra-state formulas to 600-plus area agencies on aging, the funds are so scattered that they are virtually meaningless.

Elder abuse as an issue has generated the interest of some researchers, and in the past few years there has been an increasing recognition that it shares characteristics with the dynamics of domestic violence, which has been exten-sively researched. Early studies of elder abuse focused on caregiver stress as a causative factor (ie, the older person was so difficult to care for the caregiver

---

* Corresponding author.
E-mail address: kquinn@atg.state.il.us (K. Quinn).

would "snap" and lash out through abuse and neglect) [5]. These results emerged because early studies were conducted on older persons who needed caregiving services. Later research on broader samples of older persons found that elder abuse is much a function of the characteristics of the abuser than of the victim; in fact, it much more closely resembles spouse abuse than it does child abuse [6]. Research also indicates that elder abuse victims are three times more likely to die than older persons who are not mistreated [7] and that victims of violence have twice as many physician visits and two and half times the outpatient costs compared with the general United States population [8].

Elder abuse, which affects the fastest growing population group (the aging), has yet to receive major attention at the national level. Child abuse has been a federal policy initiative for decades and receives almost $7 billion annually for services, research, training, and prevention. The abuse of younger battered women was addressed at the national level though the Violence Against Women Act in 1994, and the issue receives over $500 million in federal funds for services, awareness, criminal justice, and other professional training activities [9]. Why then does abuse of older persons, our "greatest generation," continue to be ignored?

There are several reasons. First, elder abuse had the misfortune of coming on to the national scene just as President Reagan, with his emphasis on reducing the federal government's role in social services, was elected to two terms in office, making it almost impossible to get any new social service program passed. Second, although the issue of elder abuse has attracted research and some media attention, the service system that has grown up to respond to elder abuse victims Adult Protective Services (APS) also serves younger persons with disabilities.

APS are provided in some form by every state and the District of Columbia. APS evolved out of amendments to the Social Security Act passed in 1962, which authorized states to establish protective services for "persons with physical or mental limitations, who were unable to manage their own affairs. . . or who were neglected or exploited." In 1974, Congress adopted the Title XX amendment to the Social Security Act, under which APS were an allowable expenditure. APS are now under the current Social Service Block Grant, which replaced Title XX [10].

As a result, most states passed elder abuse laws throughout the 1970s and 1980s. Because at that time the only model for state intervention into family violence cases was the child abuse system and because APS programs were created specifically for persons unable to manage their own affairs, many states adapted their child abuse statutes to address the needs of adult victims. Thus, most states enacted mandatory reporting laws for professionals who come into contact with vulnerable adults, and APS came to be criticized for being too paternalistic, especially as advocates for persons with disabilities became more organized and outspoken. To be eligible for APS help in most states, an adult has to be deemed unable to care for him- or herself. Yet, some older persons are exploited or otherwise mistreated by family members even though they are mentally and physically healthy [11].

Because each state created an APS program independently of other states and because there has been no dedicated federal funding or guidelines to encourage consistency, the result is a patchwork of laws, definitions, and services throughout the country. In some states, APS are located within the state unit on aging and the state's network of services for older people, but APS serve victims 18 and older. In other states, APS are part of the state's umbrella human services agency and may not be in the same department as the state unit on aging. In a handful of states, protective services for older persons are provided through a program in the aging network, and those same services for persons with disabilities aged 18 to 59 are provided through the human services agency. In addition, in many states, services are provided by state agencies, whereas in others they are provided by counties or by local agencies on contract with the state. Finally, all APS programs investigate cases of persons who live in the community, but many do not respond to reports in facilities [12]. The result is that the programs are hard to find, and persons who need help or want to report a case often have no idea where to go or even that such services exist.

In every case, the definitions of one state are not consistent with those of any other state. This has profound effects; for example, it impossible to know the incidence and prevalence of elder abuse in the country or even the number and type of cases reported to APS because every state defines the types of abuse differently. There are also vast differences in what types of data are collected by each state, with some states having virtually no information on their APS [12].

The result is that APS are for all intents and purposes invisible, and when attention is focused on elder abuse, APS must fight to even be recognized as the system is statutorily responsible to investigate elder abuse cases and to help elder abuse victims. Because it is so difficult to quantify the issue in a meaningful way, it makes advocating for it at the national level hard to do.

Second, elder abuse is a complex issue. Domestic violence is limited to behavior that is clearly criminal (ie, physical and sexual violence), whereas elder abuse includes neglect and financial exploitation. Much elder abuse is criminal, but a significant amount is not. A frail older spouse with osteoporosis cannot transfer a heavier spouse who has suffered a stroke; the result is that the stroke victim may be neglected and suffer serious health consequences. The frail spouse had no criminal intent and may have had the best of intentions. Intervention to protect the stroke victim is necessary even over the other spouse's objections.

Elder abuse certainly includes domestic violence, but it may take different forms than it did when the partners were younger. For example, the abuser may withhold food, water, or medicine or may refuse to take the victim to the toilet—forms of neglect that may be attributed to caregiver stress. Another example is a long-time battered woman who may neglect a now frail abusive partner.

In addition to partner abuse, domestic violence against older persons includes physical and sexual abuse by adult children, most often sons. This type of abuse may not be recognized by traditional domestic violence service systems, and a parent is usually reluctant to admit that his or her child is treating them in this way. The laws and services designed for younger battered women with small children may not meet the needs of older battered women abused by their adult sons or of older battered men.

One elder abuse case can involve multifaceted legal, medical, ethical, psychologic, financial, and family issues. A wide array of services, from orders of protection to representative payees to home-delivered meals, are needed to meet elder victims' needs. It is not enough to say "elder abuse is a crime," although it often is; the complexity of the issue may contribute to the failure to address it in a comprehensive way at the national level, especially when the service system in place serves younger persons as well.

Third, elder abuse victims are often isolated and rarely are able or willing to speak up for themselves. Children are more visible in day care or school, and younger women usually are able to flee an abusive situation. An elderly person may be confined to their home because of medical problems or because their abusers deliberately keep them there under their control. Many older victims suffer from some form of dementia, rendering them unable to seek help for themselves, or not credible when they do. The presence of cognitive problems renders elder abuse services difficult to provide.

Another complicating factor is that of self-neglect. A substantial proportion of APS cases consists of persons who are not abused by a third party but who are unable to meet their own needs [12]. Often referred to "cat ladies" or hoarders, these victims frequently have mental health problems, are resistant to services, and are time consuming and hard to work with.

In the past 10 to 15 years, there have been a number of developments in the area of elder abuse and adult protective services policies.

- Although the funding provided through Title VII of the Older Americans Act is miniscule and does not provide money for direct victim services, the recognition of elder abuse in this federal law in the early 1990s created a National Center on Elder Abuse (NCEA). The Center which has gone through two or three iterations since it was created, now consists of a consortium of six organizations: the National Center of State Units on Aging, the National Committee for the Prevention of Elder Abuse, the National Association of Adult Protective Services, the American Bar Association Commission on Law and Aging, the University of Delaware, and the Goldman Center on Aging. The Center publishes a newsletter, sponsors a national elder abuse listserv, maintains a website, conducts research and surveys, and maintains a clearinghouse of publications [13].
- The formation of the National Association of Adult Protective Services (NAPSA), originally the National Association of Adult Protective Services Administrators, the first and only national organization devoted to adult protective services as a profession. NAPSA's early years focused on information exchange, basic information collection and compilation, and training through an annual conference. One of its first accomplishments was the adoption of a policy statement by the American Association of Public

Welfare recognizing self-neglect as a form of adult abuse deserving of protective services intervention. In more recent years, NAPSA developed a statement of Ethical Principles and Best Practice Guidelines for APS. Since becoming a funded member of the National Center on Elder Abuse in 1998, NAPSA has been able to hire professional staff and to conduct national surveys of APS programs throughout the country.
- A number of efforts to get elder abuse on the national policy agenda. The 1995 White House Conference on Aging Report published several recommendations relative to elder abuse [14]; the National Institute on Aging published a research agenda on elder abuse [15]; and in 2001 the first National Policy Summit on Elder Abuse was held in Washington, DC [16], sponsored by the NCEA.

The primary goal of the 2001 Summit was to create a prioritized list of recommendations regarding a national policy agenda for protecting abused and neglected elders. Ten essential priorities were identified. NCEA listed the priorities along with an action plan on its 2002 National Action Agenda. The document was titled a "Call to Action to Protect America's Most Vulnerable Seniors."

- Priority 1 focused on urging Congress to enact a national elder abuse act. In doing so, a first-ever nationwide structure would be created to serve as a focal point for raising public awareness; funding critical services; and coordinating federal, state, and local responses.
- Priority 2 (ranking equal to the first) mandated that a national education and awareness campaign be mounted in an effort to raise America's awareness about crimes committed against older adults.
- Priority 3 set out to improve the legal landscape by strengthening elder abuse laws. It was noted that the justice system needed to take into account the special nature of elder victims and the crimes committed against them.
- Priority 4 centered on developing and implementing a national elder abuse training curriculum. The concern was that first responders, such as law enforcement, the medical community, and various domestic violence and victim/witness specialists, needed specialized training modules on systematically identifying, reporting, and treating elder abuse victims.
- Priority 5 ensured that age-appropriate and specialized mental health services were available and accessible to elders.
- Priority 6 commissioned a General Accounting Office study on how federal funds might be used. The committee wanted to know how the Social Service Block Grants were being used (as noted above, this federal block grant program to the states accounts for a significant portion of some states' APS funding).
- Priority 7 called for an increased awareness of elder abuse issues, especially within the Justice System.

- Priority 8 focused on establishing a National Institute on Aging (NIA) Research and Program Innovation Institute.
- Priority 9 was the investment in a National Resource Center on Adult Protective Services. Such a center would allow for all APS workers to have a standardized base level of knowledge and abilities.
- Priority 10 sought a Presidential Executive Order directing all federal agencies and encouraging state governors to ensure a seamless and coordinated response to all abused, neglected, and exploited seniors. Along with the order, it asked for a call for report with recommendations and findings. The impetus to create an effectively funded systematic and coordinated national response to elder abuse and neglect was derived from the 2001 Summit hosted by the National Center on Elder Abuse.

In the year after the 2001 Summit, one of the most important pieces of legislation addressing the issue of elder abuse was proposed. In 2002, Senate Bill 333, the Elder Justice Act, was first introduced into the national arena and was reintroduced in Congress in 2003 [7].

After 25 years of congressional hearings on elder abuse without serious acknowledgment of the issue, the proposed Elder Justice Act demanded that national attention be paid to the issue of elder abuse. In addition, the bill mandated that adult protective services be adequately funded. Despite the rapid growth of our aged population and the explosion of elder abuse cases, in 2004, federal expenditures directed to elder abuse by the federal government amounted to less than 1% of federal funds spent on family violence [4,7].

The Elder Justice Act (Senate Bill 333), a bi-partisan piece of legislation, reintroduced on February 10, 2003 by Senators John Breaux (D-LA) and Orrin Hatch (R-UT), set out to change the national network of underfunded, understaffed, and undertrained APS programs. An identical companion bill, H.R. 2490, was introduced in the House of Representatives by Rep. Rahm Emanuel (D-IL).

As originally drafted, the Elder Justice Act's purposes were to

1. Elevate elder justice issues to a national attention through the creation of
   (a) Offices of Elder Justice at the Department of Health and Human Services and the Department of Justice to serve programmatic, grant-making, policy, and technical assistance functions relating to elder justice
   (b) Public-private and a Coordinating Council to coordinate activities of all relevant federal agencies, States, communities, and private and not-for-profit entities
   (c) A consistent funding stream and national coordination for APS
2. Improving the quality, quantity, and accessibility of information by funding an Elder Justice Resource Center and Library to provide information for consumers, advocates, researchers, policy makers, providers, clinicians, regulators, and law enforcement and to prevent "reinventing" the

wheel. In addition, developing a national data repository to increase the knowledge base and collect data about elder abuse, neglect, and exploitation.

3. Increasing knowledge and supporting promising projects. Given the paucity of research, creating Centers of Excellence would enhance research, clinical practice, training, and dissemination of information relating to elder justice. Priorities included a national incidence and prevalence study, jump-starting intervention research, developing community strategies to make elders safer, and enhancing multi-disciplinary efforts.

4. Developing forensic capacity. There are scant data to assist in the detection of elder abuse, neglect, and exploitation. Creating new forensic expertise (similar to that in child abuse) would promote detection and increase expertise. New programs would have trained health professionals in forensic pathology and geriatrics.

5. Providing funds for victim assistance, "safe havens," and support for at-risk elders. Elder victims' needs, which are rarely addressed, would have been better met by supporting creation of safe havens for seniors who are not safe where they live and by development of programs focusing on the special needs of at-risk elders and older victims.

6. Increasing prosecution through technical, investigative, coordination, and victim assistance resources provided to law enforcement to support elder justice cases. Preventive efforts were to be enhanced by supporting community policing efforts to protect at-risk elders.

7. Training to combat elder abuse, neglect, and exploitation was to be supported within individual disciplines and in multi-disciplinary (such as public health-social service-law enforcement) settings.

8. Special programs to support underserved populations including rural, minority, and Native American seniors.

9. Model state laws and practices. A study to review state practices and laws relating to elder justice was to be performed.

10. Increasing security, collaboration, and consumer information in long-term care through
    (a) Improving prompt reporting of crimes in long-term care settings, criminal background checks for long-term care workers
    (b) Enhancing long-term care staffing
    (c) Providing information about long-term care for consumers through a Long-Term Care Consumer Clearinghouse
    (d) Promoting accountability through a new federal law to prosecute abuse and neglect in nursing homes

11. Evaluations and accountability provisions to determine what works and assure funds are properly spent [17].

Lessons learned from child welfare and domestic violence experts have taught the APS community that passage of much needed public policy must be fought for and won by the advocates. As such, the Elder Justice Coalition, a national advocacy coalition of over 100 groups and individuals who support passage of the Elder Justice Act, created a "Tool Kit for Elder Justice Advocacy Work" and disseminated the kit nationally in August of 2004. The Tool Kit provided elder rights and APS advocates with key instructions for "talking points" and other advocacy materials regarding communication with members of Congress.

The Elder Justice Coalition's efforts proved successful: 44 Senators and 91 Representatives from both parties signed on as cosponsors [17,18]. Nevertheless, the advocacy did not succeed. Although the bill was voted out of the Senate Finance Committee, after being extensively amended to reduce its scope and cost, the 108th Congress adjourned without it being called for a vote on the Senate floor. For example, the long-term care provisions, the Office of Elder Justice at the Department of Justice, and numerous other provisions were eliminated. Although funding for APS remained intact, it was scaled back to exclude services for clients under 60 years of age, although most state APS programs serve all persons with disabilities age 18 and over.

Advocates for America's vulnerable adults remain undeterred, especially because over 90% of the bill's co-sponsors will be returning to Congress. Elder Justice Coalition members have already begun to meet with key Congressional and Administration staff to discuss reintroducing the Elder Justice Act into the 109th Congress. Its scope and funding authorizations will not be known until a new bill is drafted. In addition, advocates will be active as the Older Americans Act, which provides the miniscule but now only federal funds appropriated solely for elder abuse work, comes up for reauthorization in 2005. APS and other elder justice advocates are working to use the 2005 White House Conference on Aging forum, to be held in October, 2005, to insure that elder abuse is not overlooked as an issue of critical importance to older persons in the United States.

Summary

Elder abuse remains a rapidly growing but largely invisible national policy issue. As the number of elderly persons increases, so will elder abuse, neglect, and financial exploitation. This has implications not only for the victims and the programs struggling to protect them but also for publicly funded programs such as Medicare and Medicaid. When older persons are mistreated, they require far more medical care than they would otherwise [7,8]. In addition, when someone depletes an older person's income and assets, the victim often has no choice but to reside in a long-term care facility with care funded by Medicaid, at great expense to the taxpayer. The urgent problem is to address elder abuse on a national level in a comprehensive and informed way to prevent the untold suffering of hundreds of thousands of older persons who deserve to live their final years with dignity and security.

References

[1] US House of Representatives, Subcommittee on Domestic and International Scientific Planning, Analysis, and Cooperation. Hearings of the Committee on Science and Technology, February 14–16. Washington, DC: US Government Printing Office; 1978.

[2] United States Congress. Available at: thomas.loc.gov/cgi-bin/bdquery/D?d096:26:./temp/~bdZDvt:@@@L. Accessed January 5, 2005.

[3] House Subcommittee on Health & Long Term Care of the Select Comm. on Aging. Comm. Pub. 99-516, May 10, 1985. Washington DC: US Government Printing Office; 1985.

[4] National Elder Abuse Center. Available at: www.elderabusecenter.org/default.cfm?p=laws legislation.cfm. Accessed January 5, 2005.

[5] Wolf R. Elder abuse; from aggression and violence - an introductory text. Needham Heights (MA): Allyn & Bacon; 2000.

[6] Pillemer K, Finkelhor D. The prevalence of elder abuse: a random sample survey. Gerontologist 1988;28:51–7.

[7] Lachs J, Williams C, O'Brien S, et al. The mortality of elder mistreatment. JAMA 1998;280: 428–32.

[8] Berrios D, Grady D. Domestic violence: risk factors and outcomes. West J Med 1991;155:133–5.

[9] Global Action on Aging. Breaux, Hatch introduce first ever "elder justice" bill. Available at: www.globalaging.org/elderrights/us/firstever.htm. Accessed January 5, 2005.

[10] Wolf R. The nature and scope of elder abuse. Generations 2000;24:6–12.

[11] Otto JM. Adult protective services: background, challenges, future direction and the role in abuse prevention. Generations 2000;24:33–8.

[12] Teaster P. A response to the abuse of vulnerable adults: the 2000 survey of state adult protective services. Washington DC: National Center on Elder Abuse; 2002.

[13] National Center on Elder Abuse. Available at: www.elderabusecenter.org. Accessed January 5, 2005.

[14] 1995 White House Conference on Aging. The road to an aging policy for the 21st century: executive summary. Washington DC: National Aging Information Center; 1996.

[15] Bonnie RJ, Wallace RB, editors. Elder mistreatment: abuse, neglect, and exploitation in an aging America. Washington, DC: National Academies Press; 2002.

[16] The National Policy Summit on Elder Abuse Proceedings. Washington, DC: NationalCenter on Elder Abuse; 2002.

[17] Blancato B. Elder Justice Coalition. Available at: elderjustice@verizon.net.

[18] United States Congress. Available at: www.thomas.loc.gov/cgi-bin/bdquery/z?d108:s.00333. Accessed January 5, 2005.

ELSEVIER
SAUNDERS

Clin Geriatr Med 21 (2005) 459–463

CLINICS IN
GERIATRIC
MEDICINE

Index

Note: Page numbers of article titles are in **boldface** type.

A

Abandonment, 281

Abbreviated Injury Scale, 422

Abuse, cycle of violence and, 360–361
    definition of, by different cultural
        groups, 360
    financial. See *Financial exploitation.*
    of elderly. See *Elder abuse.*

Abusers, criminal liability of, 394–395
    domineering, 284
    impaired, 284
    narcissistic, 284
    overwhelmed, 284
    recognizing and understanding of,
        283–284
    sadistic, 284
    types of, 284

Adult protective services, as community
    approach to elder abuse, 431–435
    case substantiation by, 433
    definitions of, 451
    developments in, 452–453
    history of, 431–432, 450
    interventions by, 433–434
    investigations by, 432
    myths and misperceptions about,
        434–435
    need for multidisciplinary
        collaborations, 435
    patchwork of services throughout
        country, 451
    state, 389–392

Alzheimer's disease, as risk factor for
    abuse, 288
    nursing home placement in, 289
    prognosis in, 316
    stages of, 316

Area Agencies on Aging, 444

B

Behavioral clusters, elder abuse and, 337

Bruises, as sign of physical abuse, 342

C

Caregiver, burden of, Zarit Burden Interview
    to assess, 327, 328
    depression in, 319, 320
    family, characteristics of, elder abuse
        and, 341

Caregiver stress theory, 283

Cholinesterase inhibitors, in Alzheimer's
    disease, 317

Civil liability, elder abuse and, 394
    of abusers, 394

Clearinghouse for Abuse and Neglect of the
    Elderly (CANE), 444

Code enforcement teams, 441

Cognitive decline, dementia and, 339

Community, approaches to elder abuse in.
    See *Elder abuse, community
    approaches to.*

Comprehensive Sexual Assault Assessment
    Tool (CSAAT), 402–403, 415–425
    revised (CSAAT-E), 420–421,
        422, 424

Consumer fraud, 368

Credit cards, protection of, 376, 377

Criminal liability, elder abuse and, 393–394
    of abusers, 394–395

geriatric.theclinics.com

Cultural groups, definitions of abuse
     by, 360

Cultural issues, and elder care, case illustrating,
     357–358
               family members return home and,
                    358–359
          and elder mistreatment, **355–364**

Cycle of violence, 360–361

D
_____

Deaf community, access to care, 362

Dehydration, as sign of neglect, 344

Dementia, and cognitive decline, 339
     and depression, 286
     assistance required in, 319
     care in, at home, 318–322
          in nursing homes, 322–324
     elder abuse in, **315–332**
          diagnosis of, 325–326
          treatment, intervention, and
               prevention of, 326–329
     etiologies of, 315
     medications in, 317
     progression of, losses in, 315–316
     therapies for, 316

Depression, dementia and, 286

Diogenes syndrome, 343–344

Domestic violence legislation, state,
     389–392

E
_____

Elder abuse, and neglect, **279–292**
               and exploitation, policy issues on,
                    449–457
          clues for suspecting, 341–345
          in long-term care, **333–354**
          in nursing homes, 323–324
          intervention in, 347–349
          legal definitions of, 385–386
          legal response to, 386–393
          medical implications of,
               293–313
          patient characteristics and,
               339–340
          prevention of, 346–347
          reporting of, barriers to,
               345–346
          risk factors for, 338–341
          scope of problem of, 337–338
          staff risk factors and, 340–341

as complex issue, 451–452
as criminal offense, 363
as offense, 360
background of, 279–280
behavioral clusters and, 337
by family and "friends," 383–384
characteristics of abuser and, 450
commission or omission in, 336
community approaches to, **429–447**
          adult protective services and,
               431–435
          case illustrating, 442–443
          code enforcement teams in, 441
          duty to report in, 430–431
          fatality review teams in, 441
          interdisciplinary team in, 430,
               442–443
          medical case management teams in,
               435–438, 442–443
          victim advocacy organizations,
               441–442
context of care and, 336
definition(s) of, 280–281, 334–337, 355
          based on interviews of nurses in
               nursing homes, 335–336
dementia and, **315–332**
diagnosis of, in dementia patients,
          325–326
domestic, legal and governmental
          responses to, **383–398**
          response of federal government to,
               387–388
          response of state governments to,
               388–393
facility characterisitcs and, 341
failure to report, legal actions in,
          393–394
family caregiver characteristics and, 341
forms of, 335, 356
health care professionals and, 302–303
          barriers to reporting by, 304–306
health care system use and, 298–299
health care team and, future implications
          for, 289
identification of, 285–286
ignored, reasons for, 450
in dementia patients, treatment of,
          intervention, and prevention of,
          326–329
in home, 319–320
in inability to communicate, 320
in special populations, 286–289
inattention to, 327
incidence of, 285, 317, 321
intentional or unintentional act and,
          336–337
intervention in, as controversial, 329
mortality and, 301–302
nursing home placement and,
          299–301

occurrence of, 281–282
perception of hurt and, 336
perpetrators of, legal actions against, 394–395
physical indicators of, 287
prevalence of, 384–385
preventive approach to, 327
quality of life, fear and social isolation and, 296–297
  functional decline and dependency and, 294
  self-rated health and helplessness and, 295–296
  stress and psychologic decline and, 297–298
reporters of, 285
reporting of, fear of, 361
  physicians, 294
risk factors for, 281–282, 338–341
  in long-term care, 323
screening questions, 286
strategies and interventions in, 306–308
theories to explain, 318
types of, 322

Elder Justice Act (Senate Bill 333), 454–456

Elder Law attorney, 370–371, 376

Elderly, in United States, as fastest growing segment of population, 279, 385
  sexual abuse of, studies of. See *Sexual abuse, of older adults.*
  "unbefriended," 362–363

Elderly female, sexual abuse of, forensic markers in, **399–412**

Emotional abuse, 281

Exploitation, elder abuse, and neglect, policy issues on, **449–457**
  financial. See *Financial exploitation.*

F

Fatality review teams, 441

Fear, and social isolation, quality of life and, 296–297

Financial exploitation, 281, **365–382**
  as form of abuse, 359
  cases illustrating, 365–366
  cognitive impairment as risk factor for, 320
  definition of, 367
  detection and screening protocol for, 372–373
  documentation of, 373–374

evidence of, 368
federal laws concerning, 378–379
follow-up in, 375–380
identification of, 367–369
Internet resources on, 380–381
legal aspects of, 369–372
legal definition of, 386
medical aspects of, 371–372
of older Americans, 395–396
persons perpetrating, 367
prevention of recurrence of, 378
prosecution of, 369, 370
recognition of, difficulty in, 366–367
removal of elder from situation of, 375–380
reporting of, 374–375
state laws concerning, 379–380

Forensic markers, of sexual abuse of elderly female, **399–412**

Fractures, as sign of physical abuse, 342

Fright mail, 395

Functional decline, and dependency, quality of life and, 295–296

G

Gay community, violence toward, and exploitation of, 362

H

Health, and helplessness, self-rated, quality of life and, 295–296

Health care professionals, elder abuse and, 302–306

Health care system, use of, elder abuse and, 298–299

Health care team, and elder abuse, future inplications for, 289

Health Information Portability Accountability Act (HIPAA), 432

Hygiene, poor, signs of, 343–344

L

Legal guardianship, 434

Legal intervention teams, 438–441
  civil justice system and, 440
  criminal justice system and, 439

criminal prosecution teams and,
  439–440
fiduciary abuse specialist teams,
  440–441

Long-term care, sites of, 333

Long-term care facilities, elder abuse and,
  287–288, 323, **333–354**

M

Mail fraud, 395

Medical case management teams,
  435–438
  common diagnoses of, 437–438
  history of, 436
  house calls by, 437
  interventions by, 438
  work of, 436–438

Medical neglect, signs of, 343

Mistreatment of elders. See *Elder abuse.*

N

National Center of Elder Abuse (NCEA),
  280, 285, 366, 387, 444

National Clearinghouse on Abuse in Late
  Life, 444

National Crime Victimization Survey (NCVS)
  2002, 399, 400, 410

National Elder Abuse Incidence Study
  (NEAIS), 280, 282, 429

National Policy Summit on Elder Abuse,
  453–454

Native American community, protection of
  elders by, 363

Neglect, 281. See also *Elder abuse,
  and neglect.*
  legal definition of, 386

Nursing home(s), and community settings,
  324–325
  background checks for employees of,
  349–350
  dementia in, care in, 322–324
  interviews of nurses in, definitions of
    elder abuse and, 335–336
  mistreatment in, 288
  patient neglect in, 323–324
  Pioneer Network model of care
    and, 289

placement in, elder abuse and, 299–301
    predictors of, 322
  pressure ulcers in residents of, 324
  residents of, as vulnerable, 322–323
    characteristics of, 288
  victims of sexual abuse in, 408

O

Older adults. See *Elderly.*

P

Physical abuse, 280
  legal definition of, 385–386

Physical restraints, in Alzheimer's disease, 317

Physician(s), reporting of elder abuse by, 294

Powers of Attorney documents, checking on,
  376–377

Pressure ulcers, as sign of neglect, 344–345
  in residents of nursing homes, 324

Proposed Elder Justice Act of 2003, 388

Q

Quality of life. See *Elder abuse, quality of life.*

R

Rape, prevalence estimates of, 400–401

S

Self-neglect, 281, 282–283
  legal definition of, 386
  risk factors for, 283

Senior Citizens Against Marketing Scams Act
  (SCAMS), 396

Sexual abuse, 280
  background of, 414–415
  case study of, 418–419
  criminal justice process and outcomes in,
    406–407
  of elderly, core data elements tracking,
    413–427
    incidence of, 414
    study in, 415–416
      conceptual framework of,
        416–419
      crime and case disposition
        core elements, 424–425

offender core elements and, 423–424

victim care elements and, 419–423

of elderly females, forensic markers in, **399–412**

of older adults, studies of, 401–402

   compared, 409–410

   methods of, 402–403

   results of, 403–406

offender in, characteristics of, 423

   and patterns of behavior in, 405–406

prosecution of cases of, forensic markers and, 407–408

under-reporting of, 399

victims of, forensic examination of, 405

   in community-based care, 408

   in nursing homes, 408

   mechanisms of injury to, 403–404

   patterns of injury to, 404, 405

Sexual assault, signs of, 343

Sexual Assault Nurse Examiner (SANE), 402, 410, 416

Social isolation, as sign of neglect, 345

Social Security number, protection of, 376, 377

Stress, and psychologic decline, quality of life and, 297–298

T

Telemarketing fraud, 395

U

United States Congress House Select Committee of Aging, 384–385

V

Victim advocacy organizations, 441–442

W

Women's shelters, 444

Changing Your Address?

Make sure your subscription changes too! When you notify us of your new address, you can help make our job easier by including an exact copy of your Clinics label number with your old address (see illustration below.) This number identifies you to our computer system and will speed the processing of your address change. Please be sure this label number accompanies your old address and your corrected address—you can send an old Clinics label with your number on it or just copy it exactly and send it to the address listed below.

We appreciate your help in our attempt to give you continuous coverage. Thank you.

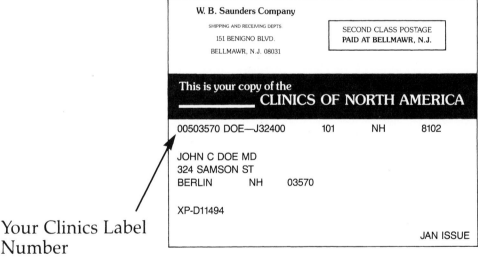

Your Clinics Label Number
Copy it exactly or send your label along with your address to:
W.B. Saunders Company, Customer Service
Orlando, FL 32887-4800
Call Toll Free 1-800-654-2452

Please allow four to six weeks for delivery of new subscriptions and for processing address changes.